Strength Training After 40

101 Exercises for Seniors to Maximize Energy and Improve Flexibility and Mobility with 90-Days Workout Plan

Baz Thompson

Strength Training After 40

101 Exercises for Seniors to Maximize Energy and Improve Flexibility and Mobility with 90-Day Workout Plan

Table of Contents

Introduction

Part One: Building Muscles

Arms

1.	Biceps Curl	12
2.	Lateral Raise	14
3.	Triceps Extension	16
4.	Lat Pull with Band	18
5.	Wall Push-Ups	20
6.	Wall Angels	22

Hands

7.	Finger Bends	26
8.	Make a Fist	28
9.	Thumb Bends	30
10.	Make a "C"	32
11.	Finger Lifts	34
12.	Wrist Stretches	36
13.	Give the Okay	38
14.	Ball Squeezes	40
15.	Assisted Finger Abductions Stretch	42
16.	Hand Open/Closes	44
17.	Thumb Flexions	46
18.	Wrist Flexion	48
19.	Wrist Radial	50
20.	Elbow Flexion	52
21.	Elbow Pronation	54

Shoulder Strengthening Training

22.	Shoulder Shrug	58

23. Kneeling Shoulder Tap Push Up 60
24. Finger Marching 62
25. Shoulder Overhead Press 64
26. Hand Grip 66
27. Skull Crusher 68
28. Forward Punches 70
29. Diagonal Shoulder Raise 72

Chest & Back

30. Chest Squeeze with Med Ball 76
31. Cat and Camel/Floor Back Extension 78
32. Renegade Arm Row 80
33. Dumbbell Bench Press 82
34. Mid-Back Extension 84
35. Reverse Flyers 86

Hips

36. Lying Hip Bridges 90
37. Side hip raise 92
38. Pelvic Tilt 94
39. Hip Extensions 96
40. Hip Abductions 98

Knees

41. Knee Extension 102
42. Squat Curl Knee Lift 104
43. Knee Curl 106
44. Knee Thrusters 108
45. Hip Marching 110

Ankle and Feet

46. Chair Stands 114
47. Toe Stand 116

Rest of the Lower Body

48. Chair Squat 120

49.	Hamstring Curls	122
50.	The Chair Dip	124
51.	Side Leg Raise	126
52.	Back Leg Raise	128
53.	Seated Marching on the Spot	130
54.	Wall Slides	132

Full-body

55.	Jog in place – warm-up	136
56.	Bird Dog	138
57.	Sit to Stand	140
58.	Good Mornings	142
59.	Calf Raises	144
60.	Bent-Over Row	146

Part Two: Stability And Balance

61.	Tai Chi 8-form	149
62.	Tai Chi 24-form	167
63.	Step Ups	216
64.	Ball Tap	218
65.	The Basic Bridge	220

Part Three: Balance And Coordination

66.	Qigong Knee Rotation Exercise	223
67.	Quadruped Opposite Arm and Leg Balance	224
68.	Rock the Boat/Balance on One Leg	226
69.	Leg Swings	228
70.	Around the Clock	230
71.	One-Legged Squat	232
72.	Single-Leg Deadlift	234

Stretches - Flexibility and Relaxation

| 73. | Chest and Arm Stretch | 238 |
| 74. | Hamstring/Calf Stretch | 240 |

75. Quadriceps Stretch — 242
76. Neck, Upper Back and Shoulder Stretch — 244
77. Standing Side Reach/Pec Stretches — 246
78. Shoulder and Upper Back Stretch — 248
79. Shoulder Rolls — 250
80. Neck Side Stretch — 252
81. Neck Rotation — 254
82. Shoulder Circles — 256
83. Shoulder Stretch — 258
84. Chest Stretch — 260
85. Overhead Reach — 262
86. Reach Back — 264
87. Triceps Stretch — 266

Water Aerobics

88. Aqua Jogging — 270
89. Leg Lifts — 272
90. Flutter Kicking — 274
91. Standing Water Push-Ups — 276
92. Arm Curls — 278

Chair Yoga

93. Overhead stretch — 282
94. Seated Cow Stretches — 284
95. Seated Cat Stretches — 286
96. Seated Mountain Pose — 288
97. Seated Twist — 290

Using Pilates

98. Mermaid Movement — 294
99. Leg Circle — 296
100. Side Circles — 298
101. Foot Slides — 300

90 Days Strength Training Exercise — 302
Conclusion — 306
References — 307

Introduction:

Do you think it is too late to build muscle and Strength after 45? Well, if your answer is a "Yes," then you might want to rethink your response in a bit!

The actual truth is that age-related changes like slower metabolism rate, shrinking of your muscle mass, and the decline of hormonal and neurological responses are bound to begin at middle age. That's precisely how our bodies are built. However, when you begin to focus on improving your fitness performance, primarily through strength training, then, believe me, magic will happen!

Working consistently and diligently towards building and maintaining your body strength comes with many beneficial packages. It helps you keep your bones healthy, thereby reducing pain from arthritis which most seniors tend to deal with as they grow older. You can also easily improve your body's mobility and stability while working your legs to prevent occasional falls and hip fractures common with older people. Being regularly active also transforms to a lowered risk of several chronic conditions and illnesses. Now you can see that exercising can be a fun and rewarding way to stay active even as a senior. Fortunately, you don't have to spend hundreds of dollars on a lengthy course to get all these benefits. This book has compiled 101 highly-effective strength training exercises that can help you reach the highest point of your fitness performance.

This book is also designed to be your ultimate guide as you begin your quest to build muscle and Strength in almost the same way younger people do. At this point, I wish you a lovely time as you read and internalize the contents of this book!

101 Workouts to Improve Balance and Stability, Restore Strength, and Enjoy an Active Lifestyle

Before getting started with any of the exercises that we will soon be discussing, let's talk about some tips that will surely help you as seniors.

Firstly, if you can afford it, you might want to get professional advice. Though most of these exercises can be performed with or without a therapist but in the most severe cases, your physical therapist must be comfortable and confident that you're able to safely do the exercises.

Staying hydrated is another necessity! Most older people tend to drink less water to avoid multiple trips to the bathroom. However, to achieve maximum results without putting yourself in danger, you must drink water before and after exercising.

In the same way, you must understand that it is impossible to out-exercise a low diet. Eating a well-balanced meal before and after a workout will undoubtedly lead to a better outcome!

Nevertheless, for every one of these exercises, having a proper form should be your primary focus. It is only by doing so that you will reap the benefits of whatever types of strength-training exercise you do.

Keep in mind that patience, determination, and consistency are vital things you must-have for this journey! Now that we have sorted the basic tips out let's get started!

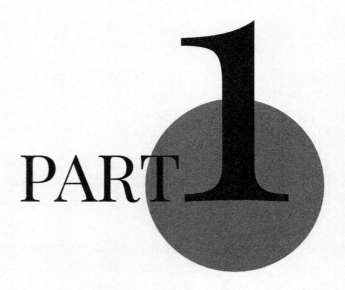

PART 1

Building Muscles

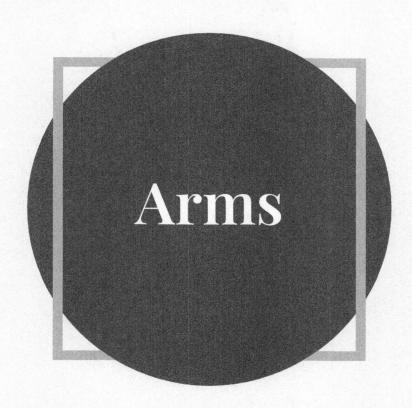

Arms

1

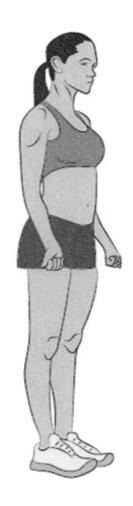 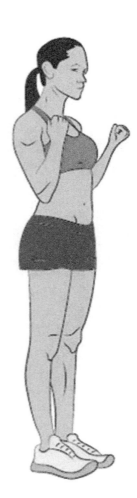

Part One: Building Muscles

1. Biceps Curl

Biceps curls are standard foundational exercises for building the muscles of the arm. By strengthening these muscles, you are also improving the stability of the motion of your arms and hands, especially when carrying anything of significance.

- Other Targeted Areas: Forearms and some of your shoulder muscles, including your deltoids.
- Length of workout: 10 minutes
- Time duration for resting periods: 30 to 90 seconds between each set.
- Estimated calorie burns: Doing about three sets of 12 bicep curl repetitions, especially with dumbbells, you are most likely to burn up to 25 calories.

Instructions:

- Get a sturdy chair and sit up tall with your hands positioned at your sides and your palms forward.
- Now focus on your arm while keeping your shoulder in; back straight, and your core tight. Focus on your biceps.
- Maintain this position and curl your arm from the elbow, all the way up to the top, and then slowly lower it back down.
- Ensure that you keep your shoulder from rotating as you completely straighten your arm on the way down and fully bend it on the way up.
- Breathing: Inhale while lifting your arm and exhale during the downward movement phase.

Level up : To make this exercise more challenging, you can hold dumbbells in your two hands and follow these instructions. For a beginner, it is recommended that you start with a two pounds dumbbell.

Precautions:

- Be gentle and don't rush as it is not how fast you are that matters. What's important is your ability to perform the movement correctly
- Go as high as comfortable.

Arms

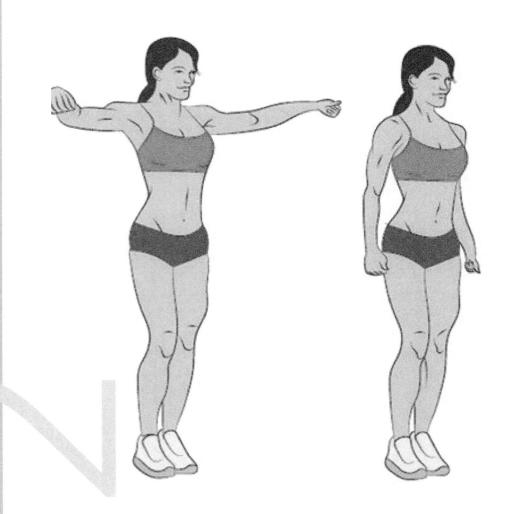

2. Lateral Raise

Upright rows are a set of upper body exercises that increase the Strength in your upper arms, thereby improving your ability to lift heavier loads.

- Other targeted areas: All your three shoulder muscles (delts, rhomboids, and teres minor) and upper back.
- Length of workout: 7 mins
- Time duration for resting periods: 30 to 40 seconds between each set.
- Estimated calorie burn: 25 calories.

Instructions

- Stand upright with dumbbells-holding hands placed in front of hips and your feet shoulder-width apart.
- While bending your elbows, lift the weights upward toward your chin.
- Make sure you do not arch the back. Keep your shoulders down.
- Return to the starting position and repeat 10 times. Rest and then go for 2 more sets.
- Breathing: inhale while lifting the weight upward and then exhale as you bring it down.

Level up: Move up to a heavier dumbbell when you feel very comfortable performing more than 20 repetitions. Or switch to an elastic band and try doing these same motion upper arms with one foot in front of the other.

Precautions

- Keep your spine straight through the movement.
- Make sure the dumbbells are not too heavy or disturbing your form

Arms

3

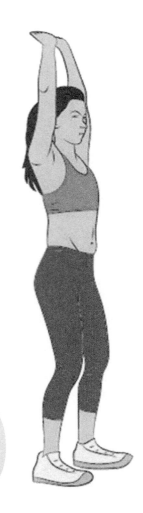
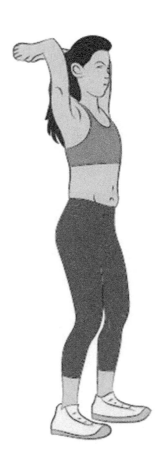

Part One: Building Muscles

3. Triceps Extension

As you've obviously detected from the name, this exercise aims to strengthen your triceps – the muscles in the back of the upper arms. The triceps muscles are involved in pretty much everything you do with your hand.

- Length of workout: 6 mins
- Time duration for resting periods: 20 to 30 seconds between sets.
- Estimated calorie burn: 16 calories

Instruction

- Sit tall in a sturdy chair with your back straight, feet flat on the floor, and legs about hip-width apart.
- Hold one hand in a tight fist, then bring your arm straight up, reaching towards the ceiling.
- Place your other hand just below the elbow of the extended arm for support.
- Now slowly lower your extended arm down and hide it behind your head.
- Bring the arm back up to the starting position. That's one rep!
- Now go ahead and do about 8-12 reps and then switch arms. To achieve effective results, aim for 3 sets of the 8-12 reps.

Level up: While these instructions are just based on your body weight, you can also go through the same motion with an extra resistance by using 1–3-pound dumbbell weights depending on your strength level.

Precautions

- Only reach your hand as high as comfortable. Pause and lower it a little bit if you begin to Precautions
- Make sure to inhale during the upward movement and exhale while lowering your hand down.

Arms

4

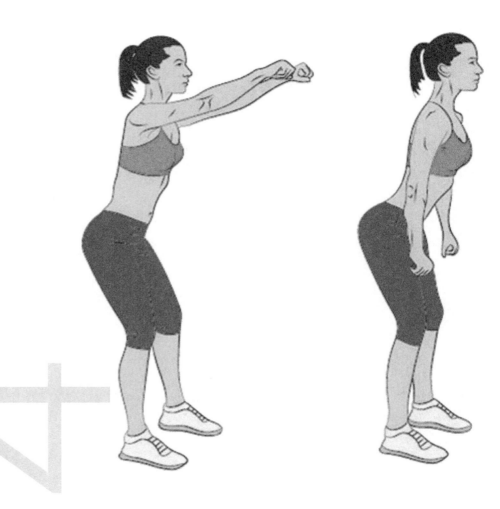

Part One: Building Muscles

4. Lat Pull with Band

Though this exercise primarily works your lats muscles on either side of the back, it also strengthens your biceps and forearms. They also provide crucial support and stability to your spine.

- Other Targeted Areas: side shoulders, back.
- Length of workout: 9 minutes
- Time duration for resting periods: 30secs -1 minutes in-between each set
- Estimated calorie burn: 36 calories.

Instructions

- Sit up and place the resistance band around your wrists.
- Raise your hands over your head in a shoulder-width position so that there is tension on the band.
- Make sure your back is flat, and your abs are engaged.
- While keeping your left hand in place, squeeze the muscles on the right side of your back to pull the elbow of your right hand down towards your rib cage. Keep it slow.
- Pause for 2 seconds and then press it back up.
- Go for 5 reps on the right side, then switch sides and do 5 reps on the left side. Go for another set of 5 reps on each side.

Precautions

- Keep your back as straight as possible throughout the movement.

Arms

5

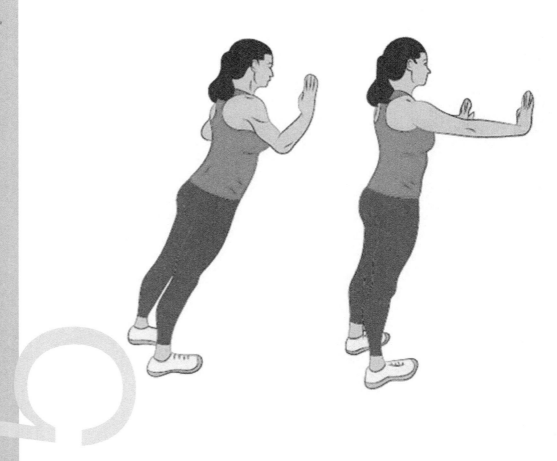

Part One: Building Muscles

5. Wall Push-Ups

- With this set of push-ups, you don't have to worry about struggling to get down on the floor and then being stuck there! Wall push-ups target and strengthen your entire upper body with a great amount of focus on your arms.
- Other target areas: Chest, back, and shoulders.
- Length of workout: 10 mins
- Time duration for resting periods: 1 to 2 minutes between sets
- Estimated calorie burn: 40 calories.

Instructions

- Get into a standing position in front of a sturdy wall, up to two feet away but as close as you need to.
- Stretch your hands directly in front of your shoulders and place them against the wall.
- Ensure that your body is in straight form. Engage your core and breathe in as you bend your elbows slowly to lean in with your chest towards the wall.
- Pause when your face is close to the wall and then exhale slowly as you straighten your arms to push your body away from the wall. That's a complete one rep
- Always remember to concentrate on this form as you go further. Keep your back and ensure that your hips don't sag.
- Go for 3 sets of 10 reps while taking rest in-between the sets.

Level up: To make the exercise more challenging, you don't really need any equipment. Just take one more step away from the wall; keep your feet shoulder-width apart, and then repeat the same motions.

Precautions

- Don't bend your elbows too much as you lean in towards the wall.
- Keep breathing properly.

Arms

6

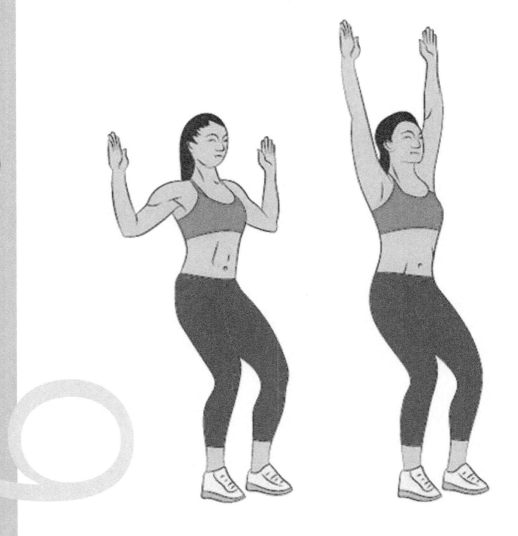

Part One: Building Muscles

6. Wall Angels

Constantly looking downwards increases tightness in your chest and middle area. What this exercise does to remedy that is to open up your chest and relieve the tension in your upper back.

- Other targeted areas: Arms, neck
- Length of workout: 6 mins
- Time duration for resting periods: 30 – 40 secs in-between each set.
- Estimated calorie burn: 25 calories

Instructions

- Stand in front of a wall with your head, lower back, and butt flat against it.
- Place your hands at your sides with the back of your palms out and against the wall.
- While keeping your arms in touch with the wall, raise them as high as is comfortable, preferably above your head.
- Slowly, bring it back down. As you go up and down, keep imagining that you're making some beautiful imaginary wings for your angel.
- Perform 3 sets of 10 repetitions.
- Try as much as possible not to lift your hips or protrude your neck during this exercise. Keep it slow!

Level up: Up for a challenge? Practice doing a hollow-sit together with the Wall Angel movement.

Precautions

- Don't place your hands too high up the wall

Arms

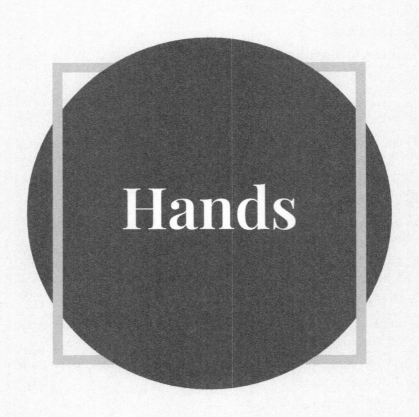

Hands

The following hand exercises will help target and strengthen your arms, wrists, fingers, and palm. But before actually performing any of these exercises, we have a good idea for warming up your hands that you don't want to miss!

It is pretty simple. Just use a microwave hot pack on your hands and palm. This will increase the temperature of the tissues, ligaments, and tendons, under your skin, making them much more elastic. Try it and see how much further and easier you can open and close your hand.

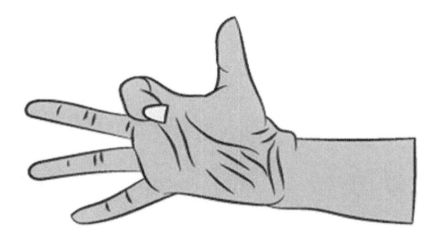

Part One: Building Muscles

7. Finger Bends

Finger Bends are a simple home exercise that keeps the joints in your fingers moving against the deterioration in hand function that is common with old age.

- Other targeted areas: Arms
- Length of workout: 8 minutes
- The time duration for resting periods: 10 secs break in-between sets
- Estimated calorie burn: 21 calories.

Instructions

- Start by holding your right hand up and straight.
- Slowly, bend your thumb down towards the direction of your palm.
- Hold the bend for two to six seconds.
- Then gently straighten out your thumb.
- Repeat the bending and releasing movement on each finger on your right hand.
- Repeat the entire sequence on the opposite hand.
- Repeat the entire movement for 4 times on both hands. Take a break and then perform another set of 4 repetitions on both hands.

Precautions

- Don't bend too hard and release the hold once you begin to feel pain

Make a Fist

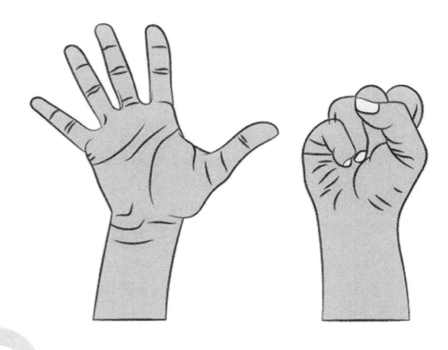

8

8. Make a Fist

The "Make A Fist" movement can help strengthen the muscles of your hands and fingers while increasing your range of motion and giving you pain relief simultaneously.

- Other targeted areas: wrist, and forearms
- Length of workout: 6 mins
- Time duration for resting periods: 10 secs in-between sets
- Estimated calorie burn: 19 calories.
-

Instructions

- Start by holding your right hand up and straight. Think of it as if you were going to give someone a "Hi-five" shake.
- Ensure that you keep your wrist and forearm close to a flat surface.
- Now, close your fingers together to make a gentle fist with your thumb wrapped across your fingers. Try not to squeeze your fingers into your palms.
- Hold that position for 10 to 30 seconds.
- Slowly release and spread your fingers wide.
- Remember to stretch only until you feel tightness. You should not be feeling pain so pause if it seems so.
- Repeat at least 5 times on both hands and then go for 3 more sets.
-

Precautions

- Release the clenched fingers when you begin to feel pain.
- Try not to squeeze your fingers too much into your palm.

Hands

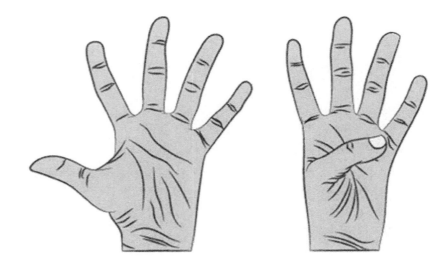

9. Thumb Bends

This exercise is just like the finger bends, except that here, we will be concentrating only on your thumbs.

- Other targeted areas: Wrist and Forearms
- Length of workout: 6 mins
- Time duration for resting periods: 10-20 secs in-between each set.
- Estimated calorie burn: 21 calories

Instructions

- Just like the previous two exercises, start by holding your right hand up and straight.
- Bend your thumb down and inward toward your palm.
- As you bend, aim to reach for the bottom of your pinky finger but still, it's okay if you cannot reach that far just yet.
- Hold the bend for 5 -10 seconds.
- Then slowly release your thumb back to the starting position. That's one rep!
- Repeat 5 times on both your left and right hand. Then go for 3 more sets!

Precautions

- Don't bend your thumbs too much to the point of pain.

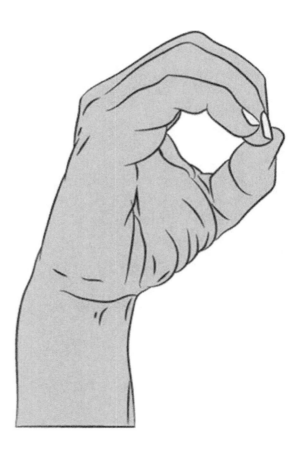

10. Make a "C"

- Length of workout: 5 mins
- Time duration for resting periods: 5 secs in-between sets
- Estimated calorie burn: 19 calories.

Instructions

- Start your right hand extended upwards and your fingers straight. To create a "C" shape, curve your fingers downward with your thumb out and to the side.
- Hold the pose for 2 to 5 seconds
- Release and Return to the starting position.
- Repeat about 10 times on your right hand
- Switch on the left hand and do 10 reps.
- Perform 3 sets of 10 reps on both hands; resting where necessary.

Precautions

- Release the hold when you begin to feel pain

Hands

11

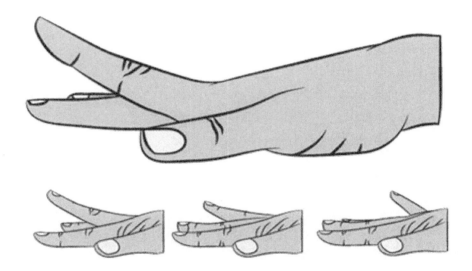

Part One: Building Muscles

11. Finger Lifts

This simple exercise helps to strengthen your hands and fingers. It also improves your flexibility and mobility level by expanding your range of motion.

- Length of workout: 8 min
- Time duration for resting periods: 10 to 20 secs in-between sets.
- Estimated calorie burn: 16 calories.

Instructions

- Start with your hand and palm-side flat on the table or any other surface.
- Slowly, lift your thumb off the table.
- Maintain that raised position for two seconds.
- Gently lower your thumb back down.
- Repeat this movement on each finger.
- Perform the entire sequence again on the opposite hand.
- Do 2 sets of 5 repetitions on both hands.

Precautions

- Only lift each finger as high as you're comfortable.

Hands

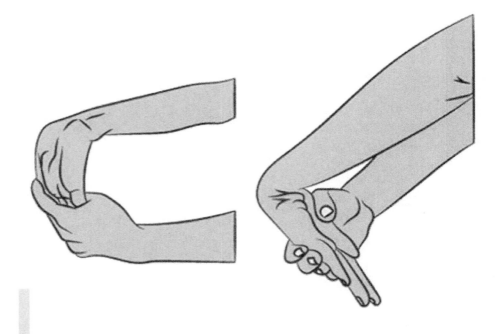

12. Wrist Stretches

Wrist pain, weakness, and stiffness are common problems for seniors. However, practicing simple wrist stretches movement is an easy and effective way to strengthen your wrists and keep your hands and fingers flexible. It also helps to lower the risk of injuries in your wrist area.

- Other targeted areas: fingers and forearms.
- Length of workout: 4 mins
- Time duration for resting periods: 10 secs in-between sets
- Estimated calorie burn: 15 calories.

Instructions

- Extend your right arm out in front of you.
- Slowly, point your fingers downwards until you feel a stretch.
- Now, use your left hand to gently pull the extended hand and finger toward your body. Hold this position for 3-5 seconds.
- Release and then point your fingers toward the ceiling until you feel a stretch.
- Use the left hand again to gently pull the raised hand toward the body. Hold this position for 3-5 seconds.
- Repeat this five times and then alternate arms
- Do 2 more sets of 5 reps on both arms.

Precautions

- Stop when you feel pain.

Hands

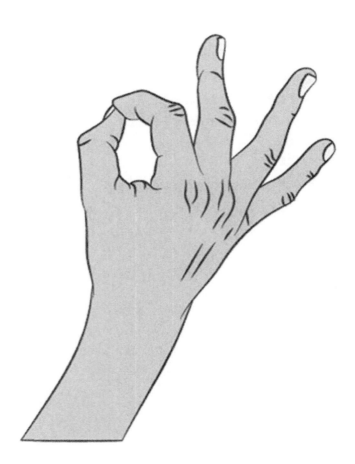

Part One: Building Muscles

13. Give the Okay

The "Give the Okay" exercise is very effective when it comes to reducing arthritis pains in your fingers. It also stretches and strengthens your finger muscles.

- Length of workout: 4 mins
- Time duration for resting periods: 5 secs before switching to the other arm.
- Estimated calorie burn: 15 calories.

Instructions

- Start with your right hand up and straight.
- Turn your thumb inwards to your index fingertip. It should create an "O" shape
- Next, touch your thumb to your middle fingertip and then repeat the same movement on the remaining three fingers.
- Go for 10-12 reps.
- Then repeat the entire exercise sequence on your left hand for the same 10-12 times.

Precautions

- Relax and pause when you feel pain.

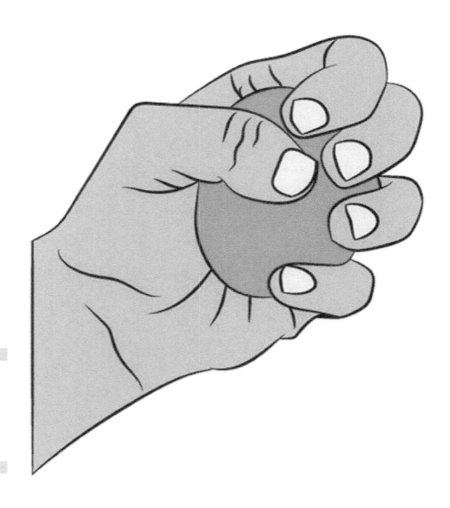

14. Ball Squeezes

Ball squeezes are simple wrist strengthening exercises that you can do while watching TV or relaxing in the garden. Asides from strengthening your grips, these stretches also help combat carpal tunnel, arthritis, and pain or weakness in your wrist and finger areas.

- Other targeted areas: Arms
- Length of workout: 3 mins
- Time duration for resting periods: 5 secs in between sets
- Estimated calorie burn: 21 calories.

Instructions

- Hold a tennis ball or just a small rubber or foam ball in your right hand.
- Slowly squeeze the ball as hard as you can and then hold it for 3-5 seconds.
- Relax the squeeze gently.
- Repeat 10 – 15 times.
- Then switch to your left hand and repeat 10 – 15 times
- Repeat 10 – 15 times more with the two hands; making it 2 sets.

Precautions

- Avoid using a very hardball at all cost
- Relax the squeeze slowly
- Assisted Finger abductions stretch

Hands

15

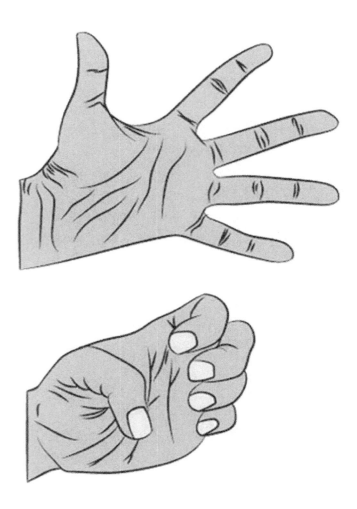

15. Assisted Finger Abductions Stretch

This exercise targets the muscles between each of your fingers which are often ignored. By stretching and strengthening them, the mobility and flexibility of the fingers eventually improve.

- Other targeted areas: Forearms.
- Length of workout: 10 mins
- Time duration for resting periods: 5-10 secs in-between sets.
- Estimated calorie burn: 15 calories.
-

Instructions

- Extend your right hand a little bit in front of you and spread your five fingers
- Use two fingers from your left hand and gently press them in between the two fingers of your extended right hand.
- Make sure that the two fingers you are using from your left hands are in scissor mode.
- You should feel the stretch as you apply a bit of resistance.
- Hold for 5 seconds and then switch to the next finger.
- Do the same for all your fingers before moving to your left hands.
- Do 3 sets of 5 repetitions.

Precautions

- If you can keep your hand steady enough, use a table for support.

Hands

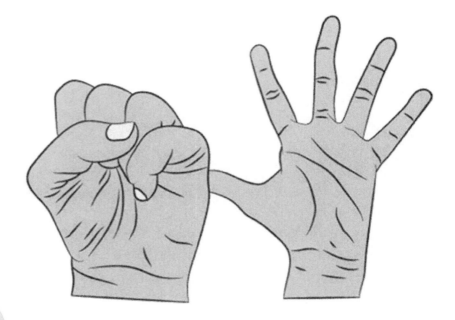

16. Hand Open/Closes

This simple exercise of clenching your fist and spreading your fingers helps to increase the Strength of your finger. It also helps to loosen up tight fingers and lowers the risk of injury.

- Other targeted areas: Forearms
- Length of workout: 4 mins
- Time duration for resting periods: 5-10secs in-between sets.
- Estimated calorie burn: 15 calories.

Instructions

- Sit with your arms extending upwards with your fingers beside your head.
- Clench your fist tight, then open up by spreading your fingers as far as you can.
- Try to make your movements as controlled and slow as possible.
- Repeat 10 times.
- Then complete 4 more sets of 10 reps.

Precautions

- Open up your hands as far as comfortable. Stop when it gets painful

Hands

17

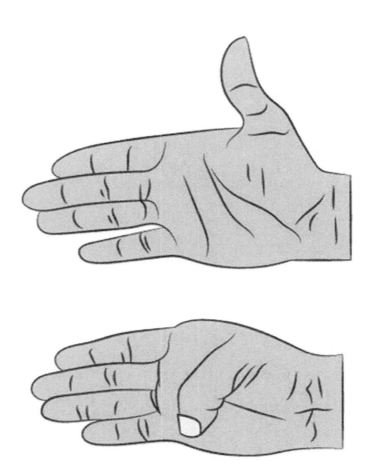

Part One: Building Muscles

17. Thumb Flexions

This exercise basically targets your thumbs. The idea here is that by working your thumb, the Strength, mobility, and flexibility in those muscles will increase.

- Other targeted areas: Arms
- Length of workout: 4 minutes
- Time duration for resting periods: 5-10 secs in-between sets.
- Estimated calorie burn: 19 calories.

Instructions

- Sit upright and extend your arms a little bit forward with your fingers spread.
- Now, slowly use your thumb to touch the tip of the index finger then open up.
- Move forward to your middle finger, close it up with your thumb and then open up.
- Repeat till you have used your thumb to touch all your other four fingers.
- You can do both hands at the same time.
- Do 2 sets of 10 reps for this exercise.

Precautions

- If you're struggling with hand joints problems, rest your hands on a table as you perform this exercise.

Hands

18

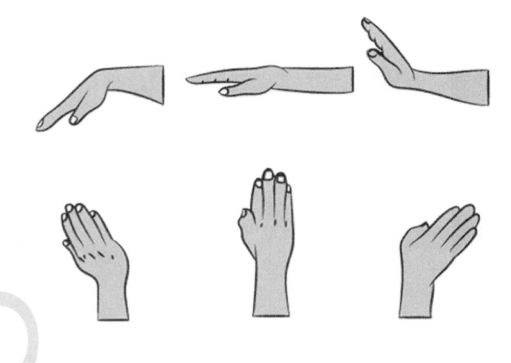

Part One: Building Muscles

18. Wrist Flexion

Wrist flexion is not just a strengthening-training exercise. It also serves as a wrist tension and pain reliever for seniors!

- Other targeted areas: Arms
- Length of workout: 5 mins
- Time duration for resting periods: 10-20 secs in between sets.
- Estimated calorie burn: 15 calories.

Instructions

- Get seated and stretch forth your right arm
- Clench your fist but make sure it is not too tight.
- Now move your wrist up and down. Keep doing that for 10 seconds.
- When you feel it too uncomfortable, you can use your other arm to support it.
- Release your fingers and then repeat the movement 5 more times.
- Switch to your other arm and do the same.
- Do 3 sets of 5 reps on each wrist.

Precautions

- Use your other arm to support your wrist as you go up and down.
- Pause and stop if you begin to feel pain.

Hands

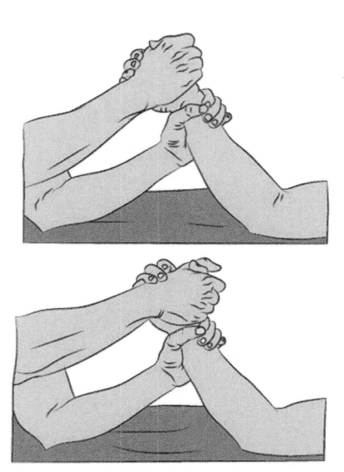

19. Wrist Radial

This exercise basically offers the same as the wrist flexion exercise. You would also see the similarities in both exercise routines.

- Other targeted areas: Arms
- Length of workout: 5 mins
- Time duration for resting periods: 10-20 secs in-between sets.
- Estimated calorie burn: 15 calories.

Instructions

- Get seated and then stretch out your arm straight with your fingers spread and your thumb facing the ceiling.
- Maintaining that position, clench your fist and then slowly move your wrist up and down for 10 secs.
- Remember to use your other arm for support. You should feel the stretch from your forearms to your wrist.
- Do 3 sets of 5 reps on each wrist.

Precautions

- Use your other arm to support your wrist as you go up and down.

Hands

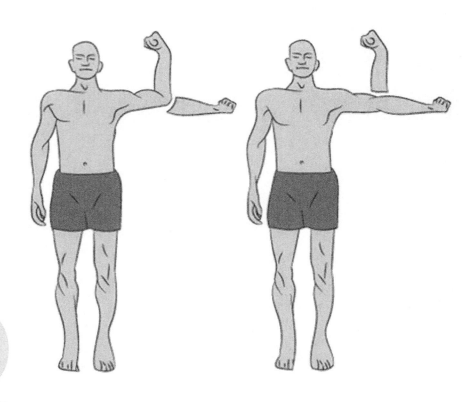

20. Elbow Flexion

Elbow flexion simply means your ability to bend your elbow. This exercise helps to expand your elbow range of motion, which in turn improves your ability to fully bend your elbows.

- Other targeted areas: Wrist and forearm.
- Length of workout: 5 mins
- Time duration for resting periods: 20 secs in-between sets
- Estimated calorie burn: 19 calories.

Instructions

- Stand up and straight with your arm at your side.
- Actively but gently bend your elbow up as far as possible.
- Then, grasp your forearm or wrist with your other straight hand and gently add resistance.
- Hold the bent position of your elbow for 5 to 10 seconds.
- Release the stretch by straightening your elbow.
- Repeat the exercise 5 times. Take a rest and then go for 2 more sets of the same 5 reps movement.

Level up: You can add a bit of stretch to your elbow flexion exercise by holding onto a 2- to 3-pound weight.

Precautions

- Be gentle as you bend your elbows
- Only go as far as you feel comfortable

Hands

Elbow Pronation

21

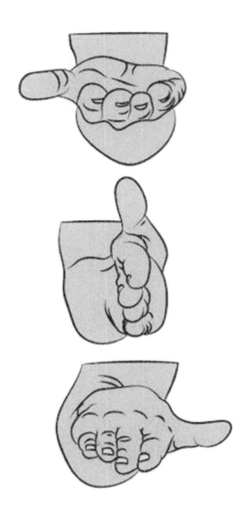

21. Elbow Pronation

Aging is associated with elbow pain which can often limit your ability to perform basic functional tasks. Being consistent with the elbow pronation exercise helps improve your ability to turn your hand over so your palm faces the floor. This motion makes it absolutely convenient for you to do tasks like pouring a cup of coffee or playing the piano.

- Other targeted areas: Wrists and forearms
- Length of workout: 5 mins
- Time duration for resting periods: 20 to 30 secs between each set.
- Estimated calorie burn: 19 calories.

Instructions

- Sit up in a sturdy chair with your elbow bent 90 degrees and tucked in at your side.
- Slowly, turn your hand and wrist over as far as possible,
- Then reach your other hand over the top of your forearm to grab your wrist, and turn your arm further into a pronated position.
- Hold the position with a little bit of resistance for five to 10 seconds. Repeat the exercise 5 times. Take a rest and then go for 2 more sets of the same 5 reps movement.

Precautions

- Only maintain the pronated position for as long as you feel comfortable.

Hands

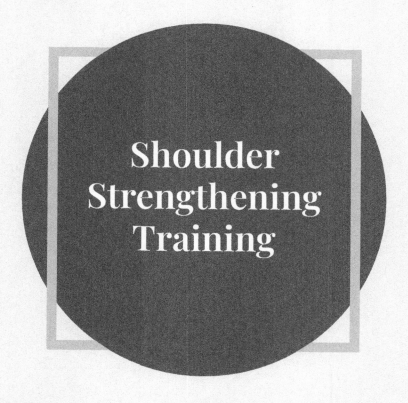

Shoulder
Strengthening
Training

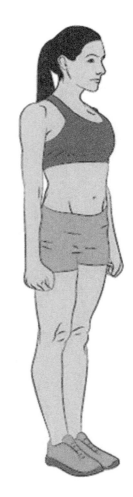
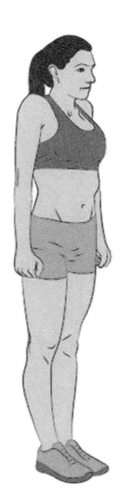

22. Shoulder Shrug

This exercise targets your scapula which is the triangle bone in the back of your shoulder. It also helps to improve the Strength, mobility, and stability of your shoulder blades. Interestingly, having a strong scapula basically translates to having functional and strong arms suitable for heavier lifting. So, let's give it a try!

- Other targeted areas: Neck and upper back muscles.
- Length of workout: 10 mins
- Time duration for resting periods: 20 to 30 secs
- Estimated calorie burn: 31 calories.

Instructions

- Get dumbbells that you are very comfortable with but try not to overdo them.
- Sit up with the dumbbells in your hands, your arms by your sides, and feet shoulder width apart.
- Now try to keep your elbows fully extended as you raise your shoulders upward slowly toward your ears. Go as high as you can, then pause for a 2-sec count.
- Exhale as you move your shoulder backward and down to return to the starting position.
- To make this motion easier, ensure that you lift your ribcage and slightly flex your knees. Also, tuck in your chin.
- Repeat 4 sets of 5 repetitions.

Level up: To take it a step more intense, try this shoulder shrug exercise while standing to increase your balance. Also, take up a heavier weight when you can perform more than 20 repetitions with no stress. Or you can switch to an elastic band.

Precautions

- Don't raise your shoulder beyond the point you feel is safe.

23

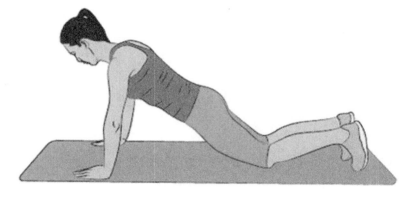

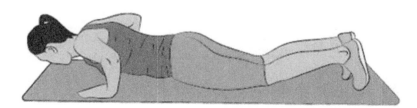

Part One: Building Muscles

23. Kneeling Shoulder Tap Push Up

This is an excellent bodyweight exercise for building muscle and Strength in the upper body. Along with targeting your shoulders, it also improves your entire body balance and stability level.

- Other targeted areas: arms, chest, back, shoulders, core
- Length of workout: 5 minutes
- Time duration for resting periods: 20 secs in-between sets.
- Estimated calorie burn: 25 calories.

Instructions

- Get into a kneeling plank position with your hands on the ground beneath your shoulders and your back extended long to the knees.
- Slowly lower your chest to the floor, keeping your core very tight.
- As you push back up to the kneeling plank position, tap your left shoulder with your right hand, then set it down.
- Repeat the push-up motion but this time, as you rise tap your right shoulder with your left hand.
- Surely, your body may want to sway side to side as you lift and lower but resist the urge to do so by keeping your core tight.
- Perform 3 sets of 4 reps each.

Level up: Switch to heavier weights.

Precautions

- Keep your core tight so that your form remains strict.
- Breathe properly in through your nose and out through your mouth.

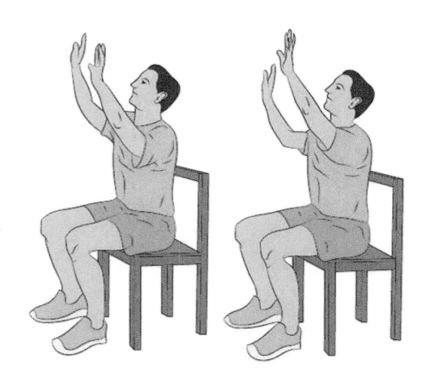

24. Finger Marching

Legs are basically for movement, but in this exercise, your fingers, hands, and arms will do the walking. The Finger Marching movement is designed to strengthen your upper body as well as improve the flexibility of your shoulders and other muscle groups close to that area.

- Other targeted areas: Arms and back
- Length of workout: 4 mins
- Time duration for resting periods: 5-10 secs in-between sets.
- Estimated calorie burn: 21 calories.

Instructions

- Get a sturdy armless chair and sit forward with your feet on the floor, shoulder-width apart.
- Now, imagine there is a wall directly in front of you. Slowly walk your fingers up the wall until your arms are extended above your head.
- Hold your wiggling fingers in that overhead position for about ten seconds and then slowly walk them back down.
- To know if you're doing this, you should be feeling a stretch in your back, arms, and chest.
- Repeat this exercise 10 times, rest, and then go for another set of 10 repetitions.

Precaution

- If you're unable to march your finger till overhead, just stop where it is comfortable and march them back down.

25

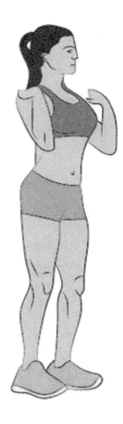
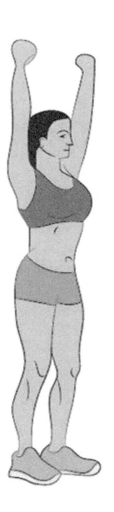

25. Shoulder Overhead Press

If you're still determined about adding size and Strength to your shoulders even as a senior, then this is another must-do shoulder-strengthening exercise that basically works your upper body to help you achieve that dream!

- Other targeted areas: biceps, back.
- Length of workout: 5 mins
- Time duration for resting periods: Rest for 20 secs in between sets
- Estimated calorie burn: 20 calories.

Instructions

- Start with dumbbells in your hands and your feet hip-distance apart.
- Now stretch your elbows out to the side creating a goal post position with arms.
- Your dumbbells-holding hands should be at the side of the head, and the abdominals are tight.
- Slowly lift the dumbbells until the arms are straight. Pause for two seconds.
- Then with the same level of control, return to the starting position with control.
- Repeat this exercise 5 times, rest, and then go for 2 more sets.

Level up: Switch to heavier dumbbells.

Precautions

- Only raise your arms as high as comfortable.
- Keep your core tight.

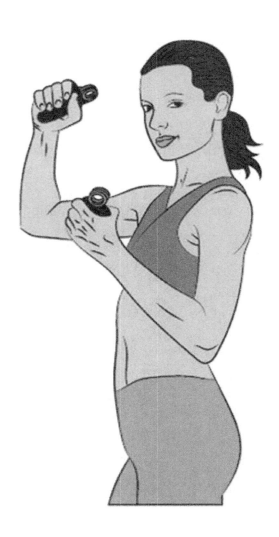

Part One: Building Muscles

26. Hand Grip

Usually, your grip strength tends to decrease as you age. Thus, this exercise is specifically designed to increase your grip strength, dexterity, and flexibility in your hands and fingers. The hand grip movement can make it easier for you to open door knobs and hold things without dropping them. It is very safe for seniors of any age and grip strength level.

- Other Targeted Areas: Forearms
- Length of workout: 6 mins
- Time durations for resting periods: 10 - 20 secs in-between each set
- Estimated calories burnt: 21 calories.

Instructions

- Grip a soft stress ball in your palm and squeeze it as hard as you can comfortably.
- Hold for 5 - 10 seconds and then release.
- Complete 3 sets of 5 to 10 reps on each hand.
- Level up: To add intensity, you can switch to using a firmer stress ball when using the soft stress ball becomes easier.

Precautions

- Make sure you warm up your hands before exercising them. This is because this hand grip exercise can lead to finger and wrist strain if the muscles aren't stretched first.
- Totally avoid this exercise if your thumb joint is damaged.

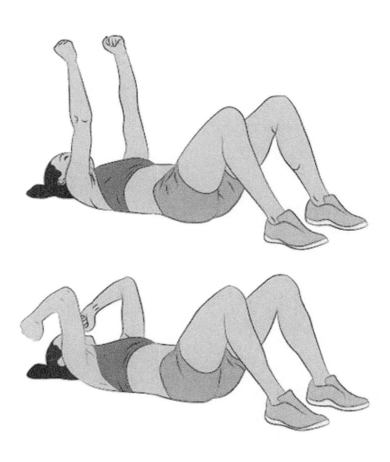

27. Skull Crusher

The skull crusher movement is an isolation exercise that targets and builds your triceps muscle group. It also helps in fixing imbalances with the triceps without you having to place pressure on your wrists. Just so you know, the name "skull crusher" originates from the fact that if you use poor form, you could endanger your skull. Hence you have to be extra careful with it.

- Other Targeted Areas: Upper Arms.
- Length of workout: 7 mins
- Time duration for resting periods: 30 - 40 secs in-between each set.
- Estimated Calories burnt: 27 calories.

Instructions

- Get a flat gym bench and lie on it with your face up and your legs comfortably placed to each side on the floor.
- Hold the dumbbell tight and straight up with both hands above your chest and the dumbbell shaft in a vertical position. Make sure your elbows are not locked.
- Now inhale and slowly move the weight down toward the rear of your head by flexing your elbows while exhaling.
- Only elbows should be moving here, so keep your upper arms from moving back and forth with the weight.
- Continue to lower the weight behind your head until the dumbbell head is about in line with the bench top.
- Slowly reverse the movement to the point where the weight is held above the chest. And you've just completed one rep!
- Repeat 5 to 8 times for each of two sets.
- Level up: If you're up for a challenge, try performing this same movement on an inclined bench.

Precautions

- Your starting position should be stable and comfortable.
- Don't lower the weight toward the face or forehead. Instead, ensure that it passes over your head
- Take care not to hit the back of your head when raising the dumbbell from behind the head to return to the starting position.
- This exercise should be done slowly and carefully under good control.

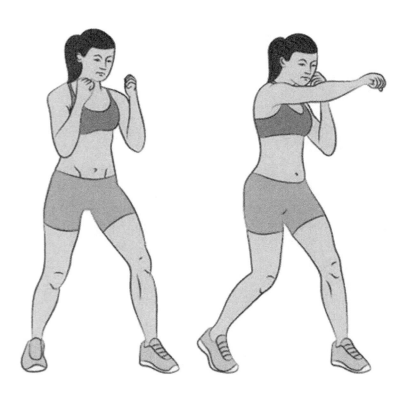

28. Forward Punches

This is a warm-up exercise that you can use to strengthen your shoulder and arms,

- Other targeted areas: Arms
- Length of workout: 10 mins
- Time duration for resting periods: 20-30 secs in-between sets.
- Estimated calorie burn: 59 calories.

Instructions

- Get seated and make fists with your hands. Hold them in front of your chest at shoulder height.
- Envision a punching bag out just at arm's length. Then bring one arm forward to punch it and then return it.
- Alternate and bring the other arm forward and return.
- Make sure that you keep your abdominal muscles tight as you punch.
- Repeat 20 times and complete 5 sets.

Level up: Use water bottles or small hand weights to make the workout more challenging.

Precaution

- Ensure that you don't punch extremely hard so as not to get problems in your upper arms.

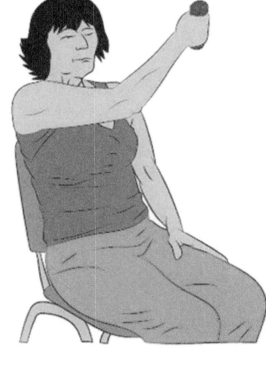

29. Diagonal Shoulder Raise

This shoulder strengthening exercise is a multi-beneficial one for seniors. It helps to improve your shoulder muscle size, function, and neural control. It is also a great tool for fighting and defeating osteoporosis.

- Other targeted areas: Arms
- Length of workout: 5 mins
- Time duration for resting periods: 10-20 secs in-between sets.
- Estimated calorie burn: 45 calories.

Instructions

- First, sit with a dumbbell in your hand. Your hand should be over your opposite hip with your palm facing inward.
- Next, lift your arm up and across your body to the side. By this time, your palm should be outward.
- Then go back to the start position and do ten repetitions. That's the Diagonal Outwards Shoulder Raise.
- For the inward movement, your palm should be forward,
- Now lift your arm up and across your body to the opposite shoulder. Bend your elbow as you bring your arm over and face your palm inward. Repeat ten times.
- Switch to your other arm and do the same.
- Take a rest and then go for one more set on each hand.

Level up: Switch to heavier weights when you can perform 20 reps easily.

Precautions

- Avoid over-bending your elbows.
- Keep the movements slow.

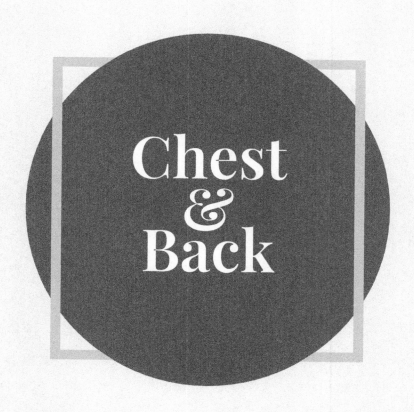

Chest
&
Back

30

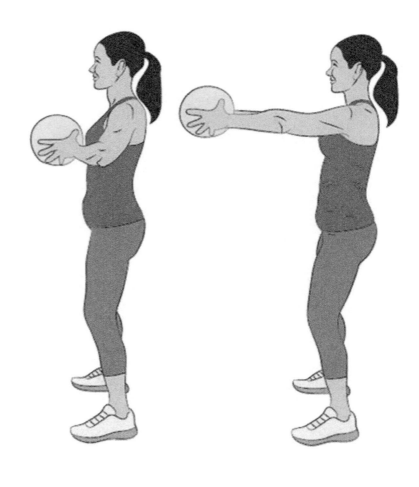

30. Chest Squeeze with Med Ball

At this point, you will notice that the exercises are getting more intense. But trust me, they are still totally easy and fun for seniors of varying fitness levels. This chest squeeze movement is excellent for building and strengthening your chest muscles. Essentially, you're going to need a medicine ball for this to help improve your balance and stability. If you're a beginner in this game, then a good starting point will be around 6 – 8 lbs for older females and 8 -15 lbs for older males.

- Other targeted areas: Arms and glutes.
- Length of workout: 5 mins
- Time duration for resting periods: 20 – 30 secs in-between sets.
- Estimated calorie burn: 48 calories.

Instructions

- Get seated in a sturdy chair with your back straight and feet flat on the floor.
- Tighten your core as you hold the ball with both hands.
- Lift your arms to your chest level by making your elbows bent and out to the sides. Your forearms should be parallel to the floor.
- While putting even tension on the ball with both hands, and squeezing your chest, push the ball forward till your elbows and arms are completely straightened.
- Then pull the ball back to your chest, by bending your elbows.
- Complete 3 sets of 5 reps; resting when necessary.

Level up: To make it more intense, you can wrap a resistance band around your back, with your thumbs/palms at each end of it as you push and pull the medicine ball at your chest level.

Precautions

- Try not to use the Med Ball to hit your chest.
- Use the appropriate weight for your strength level.

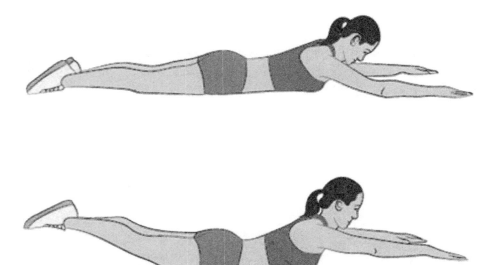

31. Cat and Camel/Floor Back Extension

This is a beginner's stretch that you as a senior will be able to do relatively easily. The cat and camel movement stretch and strengthens your back and abdominal muscles. Thus, giving you the chance to regain or improve your ability to turn and maneuver in your daily activities without the fear of losing your balance.

- Other targeted areas: Abdominal muscles, hips.
- Length of workout: 4 mins
- Time duration for resting periods: 5-10secs in-between sets.
- Estimated calorie burn: 20 calories.

Instructions

- Get on all fours, either on a yoga mat, bed, or another soft surface, with your back straight, hands shoulder-width apart, and your fingers facing forward. Your back should also be straight and knees a few inches apart.

- While keeping your abs tight, slowly and gently begin to arch your back and lift your head so that your eyes are looking upwards. That's the cat pose.

- For the camel pose, curve your back upward and lower your head downward. You should feel the stretch in your spine.

- Breathe in when you arch your back down and exhale as you curve your back up. That's one complete rep

- Do 2 sets of 5 reps.

Precaution

- Stop the exercise immediately and you begin to feel pain in your spine.

32

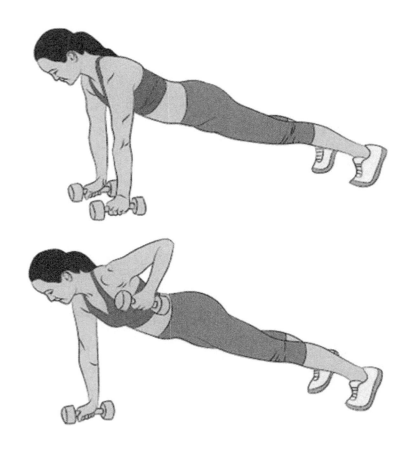

32. Renegade Arm Row

This exercise is an upgrade from the bent-over row and upright row. It targets almost every part of your upper body as well as your core. The renegade arm row also highlights any imbalances in your upper body and eventually helps in stabilizing the targeted areas.

- Other targeted areas: Arms, abdominal muscles, shoulders.
- Length of workout: 8 mins
- Time duration for resting periods: 30 – 60 secs in-between sets.
- Estimated calorie burn: 56 calories.

Instructions

- Grab a pair of light dumbbells and get into a press-up position with the dumbbells in each hand.
- Tighten up your abdominal muscles, as you slowly raise your left dumbbell-holding hand while supporting yourself on the other arm.
- Row the dumbbells upwards till it reaches slightly above your torso.
- Still keeping that control, slowly lower the weight back to the ground.
- Repeat 5-6 times and then switch to the other side.
- Keep breathing in through your nose as you lift your arm and out through your mouth as you lower it to the ground.
- Perform 3 reps of 5-6 repetitions on each side.

Level up: Switch to a heavier weight when you are sure you are ready for the challenge.

Precaution

- Opt. for a lighter dumbbell that is fit for your strength level. Do not overestimate.
- Keep your movement slow and steady.
- It is okay if you cannot raise the dumbbells above your torso; just make sure you go only as high as comfortable.

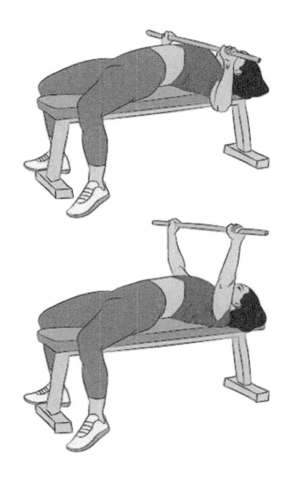

33. Dumbbell Bench Press

This superb compound movement works on your chest muscles to help build enough muscular Strength there. For the fact that it doesn't really require balance, the bench press exercise is one of the safest exercises for seniors especially those with knee problems. However, it is not recommended for those with shoulder pains.

- Other targeted areas: Shoulders, Triceps and Biceps.
- Length of workout: 15 mins
- Time duration for resting periods: 3 minutes in-between each set.
- Estimated calorie burn: 111 calories

Instructions

- Choose a dumbbell that is heavy enough for you to do 12 – 15 reps comfortably but not too comfortably
- Now, lie flat on your back; on a bench, with your feet flat on the ground.
- With a dumbbell in each hand, slowly extend your arms directly above your shoulders, palms facing toward your feet.
- To lower the weights down, squeeze your shoulder blades together and slowly bend your elbows until it is parallel with your shoulders, forming 90-degree angles.
- With the same controlled slow motion, drive the dumbbells back up to start, making sure to squeeze your shoulder blades the entire time. And you have one complete rep!
- Repeat for five to six reps, performing three sets afterward.

Level up: If you're sure that you are fit to take it up a notch, then try the bench press with an Olympic unloaded bar or seated chest machine.

Precautions

- Don't over-squeeze your shoulder blades.
- Rushing with your movement will only increase your injury risk so do them slowly.

34

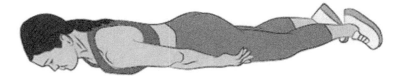

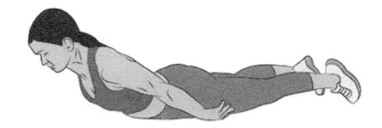

34. Mid-Back Extension

This exercise is also known as the prone cobra movement. It basically focuses on stretching, extending, and strengthening your lower back and mid-back muscles, making it easier for you to maintain good posture when sitting or standing. It can also help to relieve mid back pain associated with postural strain.

- Other targeted areas: Neck, Arms
- Length of workout: 7 mins
- Time duration for resting periods: 30 – 40 secs in between each set
- Estimated calorie burn: 32 calories

Instructions

- Start by lying face down on your bed or the floor with your hand and palm down by the side of your face. For comfort, you may place your forehead on a rolled-up hand towel.
- Slowly pinch your shoulder blades together and lift your hands off the floor. Your shoulder should be down and away from ears
- Roll your elbows in with your palms out and thumbs up.
- Gently lift your forehead about an inch off the towel but keep your eyes looking straight at the floor and not forward.
- Try to hold that position for 10 seconds.
- Make sure that you maintain your hips on the floor and don't hold your breath. Keep breathing in through your nose and out through your mouth.
- Return to the starting position and repeat 5 times. Take a rest and go for two more sets.

Level up: To increase the intensity of the exercise slightly, you can also lift your legs off the ground.

Precautions

- Keep your movement very slow and controlled

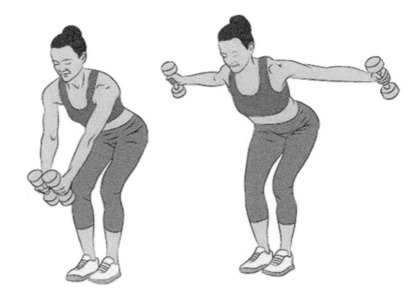

35. Reverse Flyers

The reverse fly is a resistance exercise that targets the major muscles of the upper back, including the trapezius. This exercise helps to improve your stamina by strengthening these muscles that are usually negatively affected by poor posture.

- Other targeted areas: Neck, Rear shoulders, and upper back
- Length of workout: 10 mins
- Time duration for resting periods: 30 – 40 secs in-between each set.
- Estimated calorie burn: 36 calories.

Instructions

- Stand upright with your arms holding dumbbells at the sides and feet shoulder-width apart
- Slowly, press your hips back in a hinge motion bringing your chest forward almost parallel to the floor.
- Allow the weights to hang straight down, as you maintain a tight core, straight back, and slight knee bend.
- Breathe out and raise both arms out to your side, squeezing the shoulder blades together.
- Bend your elbows a little bit as you pull your shoulder blades toward the spine.
- Now, take in a deep breath as you lower the weight back to the starting position.
- Avoid hunching your shoulders up during the movement, instead, keep your chin tucked and focus on feeling the shoulders blades coming together.
- Repeat the exercise for 4 times for 3 sets.

Level up: Increase weight resistance during the exercise by lifting heavier dumbbells.

Precautions

- Don't ignore the breathing rules.
- Keep your shoulder back throughout the movement.

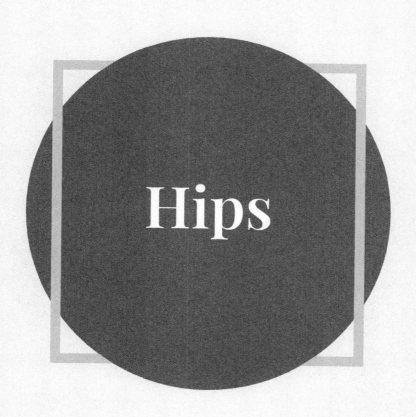

Hips

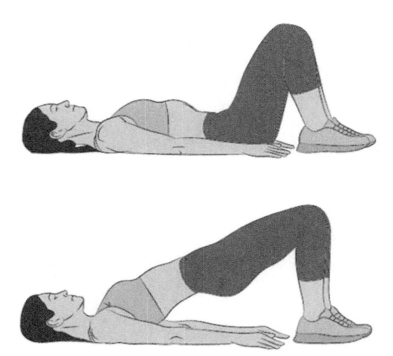

Part One: Building Muscles

36. Lying Hip Bridges

Lying hip bridges is one of the most important strength-training hips exercises for seniors. It targets and works your body's largest muscle group, which is the glutes; your butt muscles. Fortunately, it starts and ends with you lying on your back.

- Other targeted areas: Abs, hamstrings, lower back
- Length of workout: 7 mins
- Time duration for resting periods: 20 - 30 in-between each set.
- Estimated calorie burn: 32 calories

Instructions

- Lie on your back with your hands by your side, knees bent, and feet flat on the floor.
- Flatten your lower back against the floor, to tighten your abdominals and squeeze your butt muscles, then lift your hips into the air to create a straight line from your knees to shoulders.
- As you lift your hips, push through your feet.
- Hold for 10 to 15 seconds, and then slowly lower your hips and return to your starting position.
- Complete 2-3 sets of 10 reps.

Level up: Use a resistance band to bind your legs and follow these same instructions. You will surely find it more intense.

Precautions

- Lower your back to the ground once you begin to feel pain. You don't have to hold the hip bridge pose for up to 15 seconds.

Hips

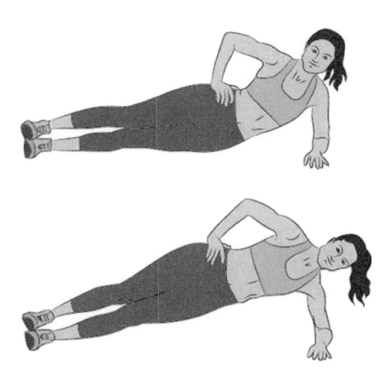

37. Side Hip Raise

The exercise is an exceptional hip arthritis-relieving exercise that delivers great results for seniors and the elderly. It minimizes your pains and safely strengthens your side hip muscles.

Performing it correctly and consistently will also help improve your lower body endurance so that you can easily walk and sidestep around objects.

- Other targeted areas: Lower back muscles and glutes.
- Length of workout: 4 mins
- Time duration for resting periods: 10 -20 secs in-between each set.
- Estimated calorie burn: 25 calories.

Instructions

- Stand upright and hold on to a sturdy chair to balance yourself.
- Lift your right leg to the side as high as comfortable and pause for a 2 secs count. Lift your ribs too!
- Try not to bend at the hips; stand as straight as possible.
- Return to the starting position, then repeat 5 times and switch to the left leg.
- After completing that, go for one more set of 5 reps on both legs.

Level up: To increase the intensity of the workout, try holding on to the chair with just one hand, then one finger, and eventually let go completely to balance on your heels. You may also add a 2 to 5-pound ankle weight to your leg.

Precautions

- Keep your body erect and breathe properly
- Don't lift your hips too high.

Hips

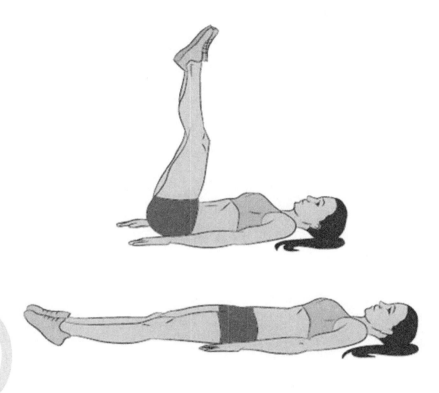

Part One: Building Muscles

38. Pelvic Tilt

The pelvic tilt exercise is a stretch and strength-building movement combined. It is beneficial for releasing tight hips caused by prolonged sitting. It also helps to increase the range of motion and flexibility of the pelvic region.

- Other targeted areas: Core and lower back.
- Length of workout: 6 mins
- Time duration for resting periods: 30 seconds to a minute between each set.
- Estimated calorie burn: 25 calories.

Instructions

- Lie on your back, whether on your mat or bed with your knees bent and feet flat on the ground.
- Tightening abdominal muscles, push your lower back into the floor. Release a deep breath while letting your hips and pelvis also rock back.
- Hold this position for five seconds, then relax with your lower back rising off the ground slightly.
- Make sure to inhale as you relax.
- Repeat 2-3 sets of 5 reps.

Level up: Combine this pelvic tilt exercise with alternating arm raises to take it up a notch!

Precaution

- Keep your spine straight as you lower your back

Hips

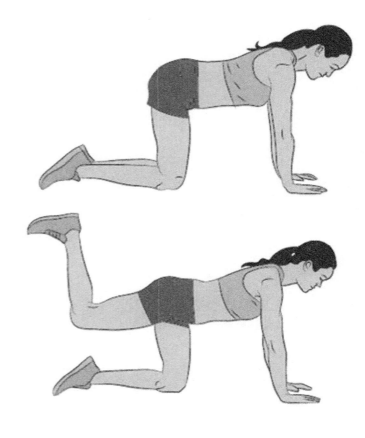

Part One: Building Muscles

39. Hip Extensions

These hip extension exercises target and strengthen your legs, and hip flexor muscles. Strengthening these muscles will, in turn, improve your balance and assist in walking and standing. Before you know it, you will be propelling yourself forward or up the stairs easily and without any help.

- Other targeted areas: Glutes, hamstrings.
- Length of workout: 4 mins
- Time duration for resting periods: 10 -20 secs in-between each set.
- Estimated calorie burn: 25 calories

Instructions

- Stand upright, using a chair to balance yourself.
- Tighten your tummy muscles and keep breathing as you slowly extend your left leg backward. Keep your body erect and your knee straight.
- Pause a little, then gently lower your leg back to the ground to return to the start position
- Repeat 2 sets of 10 reps with each leg.

Level up: For a more challenging workout, add a 2 to 5-pound weight to your ankles. But first, try using a single hand, one finger, or no hands to balance yourself.

Precautions

- If you have knee problems, use two chairs instead of one for support.

Hips

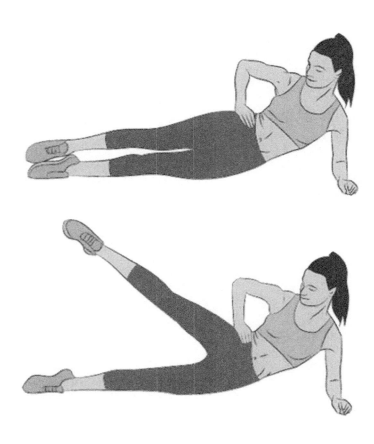

40. Hip Abductions

This exercise aims to build and strengthen your hip abductors. It also trains your lower body to provide core stability, build balance, and good posture.

- Other targeted areas: abdominals, back muscles, buttocks (glutes).
- Length of workout: 5 mins
- Time duration for resting periods: 20 - 30 secs in-between sets
- Estimated calorie burn: 29 calories.

Instructions

- Standing tall with your feet close together and hold on to a sturdy chair.
- Your hip, knee, and foot should be pointing straight forward with your body erect
- Slowly lift your leg out to the side and in a controlled motion bringing your feet back together.
- Pause for 3-5 secs. Make sure that you do not lean or hitch your pelvis during this pose.
- Gently return to the starting position.
- Repeat for 2-3 sets of 4 repetitions on each leg.

Level up: Place a resistance band around both your legs at the thigh level.

Precautions

- Try not to hitch your pelvic throughout the movement.
- Never hold your breath.

Hips

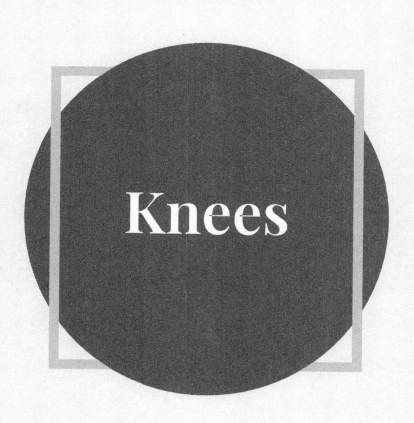

Knees

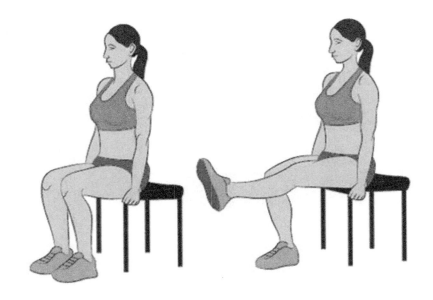

Part One: Building Muscles

41. Knee Extension

The ability to stand easily and fully extend your knee is very vital for every human being. Unfortunately, aging causes the knee joints to lose some of their flexibility and range of motion. That's why this knee extension exercise aims to strengthen your knee joints, thus improving your ability to stand and balance as well as your available knee range of motion.

- Other targeted areas: Quadriceps (Thighs)
- Length of workout: 6 mins
- Time duration for resting periods: 30 - 40 secs in-between each set.
- Estimated calorie burn: 31 calories.

Instructions

- Sit up tall in a chair with your feet flat on the floor and your shoulders back and down.
- Slowly lift your leg up and extend the knee.
- Hold for a few seconds when you have fully straightened that knee. At the same time, try squeezing the muscles at the front of the thigh.
- Next, slowly lower your leg back down and alternate your legs.
- To use your full range of motion, ensure to bring your heel fully back as far as comfortable then extend.
- Repeat for 3 sets of 5 reps and rest where necessary

Level up: To take this exercise a step higher and accelerate your strengthening, add ankle weights to your ankle.

-

Precautions

- Using immense control, move your leg slowly without jerking it.
- Do not hold your breath. Inhale as you lift your leg and exhale as you lower it back to the ground.
- Your back should remain straight against the chair, so no slouching!

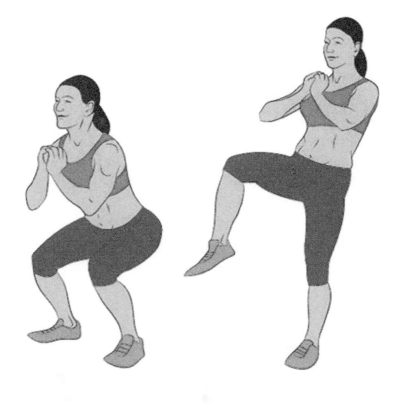

Part One: Building Muscles

42. Squat Curl Knee Lift

Of course, the combination of three individual exercises into one will definitely seem intimidating if not totally impossible especially for seniors. But you don't have any cause to worry since the squat, curl and knee lift movements are all super basic and easy to learn if you haven't tried them out already. This multitasking strength training exercise works a lot of different muscles all at once with a major focus on your knees and quads. It is also a very reliable way to help lessen the symptoms of the following chronic conditions like arthritis and osteoporosis. Another great thing is that all you need is a pair of dumbbells.

- Other targeted areas: biceps, glutes, quads.
- Length of workout: 10 mins
- Time duration for resting periods: 30 secs - 1 minute in-between each set.
- Estimated calorie burn: 28 calories.

Instructions

- Start in a squat position with your chest lifted, shoulders down, and abs tight.
- Weight back on your heels with your arms straight next to your side, holding dumbbells.
- Squeeze your glutes to press upwards and lift your right knee as you curl the weights to your shoulders.
- When you curl, ensure that your elbows are as close to your body as you can.
- Now, lower the dumbbells back down and return to your squat position. Then repeat with the left knee.
- Perform 2-3 sets of 5 reps per side.

Level up: Switch to heavier dumbbells.

Precautions

- Make sure to choose weights that can create enough resistance for your biceps to feel the burn. However, ensure that it is not at the expense of you losing your form or feel any form of pain.
- Do not rush with this movement; just keep your movement slow and well-controlled.
- Do not let your knees go over the toes too far as that can place excessive pressure on your knee joints.

Knees

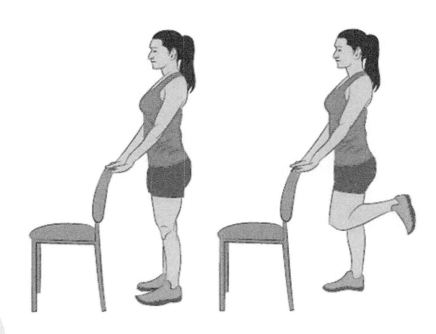

43. Knee Curl

This exercise is an ideal exercise for you as a senior to improve your leg strength and balance. Kneel curls strengthen your hamstring muscles and having stronger hamstrings, in turn, helps in strengthening your knee joints. It also improves their flexibility and balancing abilities

- Other targeted areas: Hamstring muscles
- Length of workout: 10 minutes.
- Time duration for resting periods: 40 secs - 1-minute in-between sets.
- Estimated calorie burn: 31 calories.

Instructions

- Get a sturdy chair and stand upright with your front-facing it.
- Space your feet hip-distance apart as you hold the back of the chair to maintain your balance and for support.
- Shift your weight onto your left leg and slowly bend your right knee, bringing your heel up toward your buttocks as far as possible.
- Hold this position for 1-3 seconds. Make sure your hips remain still and thighs parallel. The left leg you are standing on should also be slightly bent.
- Now, slowly lower your right foot back down to the ground. Go for 8 - 10 reps on your right leg.
- Then switch to your other leg for the same amount of reps. This will complete one set. Aim for 2-3 sets.

Level up: If you're up for a challenge, perform the same motions without holding the back of the chair for balance.

Precautions

- Ensure that you do not arch your back as you lower and lift your leg.
- Keep your movements slow and controlled without any jerks. Rushing will only result in injury.

Knees

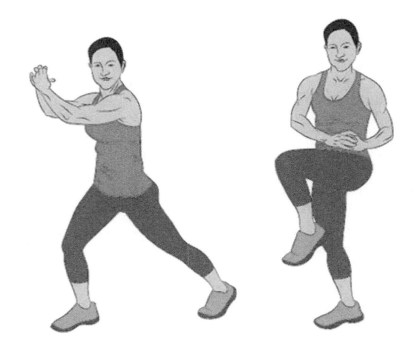

Part One: Building Muscles

44. Knee Thrusters

Knee thrusters are great low-impact exercises that strengthen your lower body and core while getting your heart rate up. This in turn helps in improving your pelvic stability. The idea here is that you're visually crushing something against your knee

- Other targeted areas: hip flexors, back muscles, core (abdominals), triceps, shoulders
- Length of workout: 5 mins
- Time duration for resting periods: 20 -30 secs in-between each set.
- Estimated calorie burn: 25 calories.

Instructions

- Get into a standing position with your feet wider than shoulder-distance apart.
- Turn both feet in one direction, allowing your hips to follow in the same direction like you're doing a shallow lunge.
- The front knee should be at a 90-degree angle with the back heel lifted. Also, extend your arms up in a guard position in front of the chest.
- Lift your back knee up to your hip height toward the hands, then lower your hands in toward the thigh.
- Return the foot to the floor. Repeat 6-8 times and then alternate legs.
- Complete 2-3 sets of 6-8 reps on each leg.
- Level up: To add more resistance, you can use a resistance band around your knees.

Precautions

- Keep your movement slow, controlled and smooth.

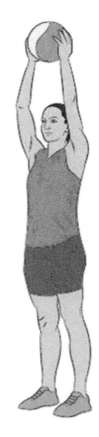
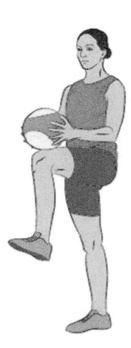

45. Hip Marching

The hip marching exercise is designed to strengthen your hips and knees. By doing this, this movement also improves your walking endurance and ability to bend pick up objects off lower surfaces.

- Other targeted areas: thighs, abdominal muscles.
- Length of workout: 7 mins
- Time duration for resting periods: 30 -40 secs in-between each set
- Estimated calorie burn: 21 calories

Instructions

- Sit in a chair with your feet flat on the floor and your back straight against your back.
- Slowly, lift up your right knee as high as comfortable.
- Hold the position for one second and then gently lower your leg.
- Alternate lifting your knees for 5 reps on each leg, then rest and go for one more set.

Level up: Place your hands on your thighs and resist the upward movement of your knees by pushing downward.

Precautions

- Move at a slow to moderate speed and continue breathing throughout the exercise.
- No matter how strong you might feel, don't perform more than 20 hip-marching moves in a row. That is your best option to avoid fatigue and soreness.

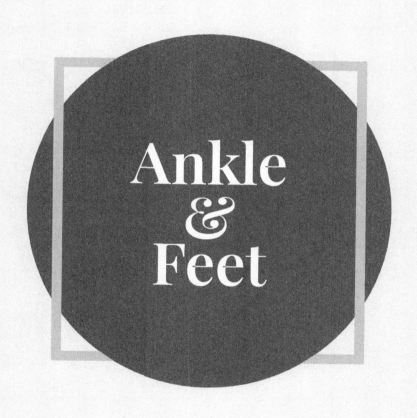

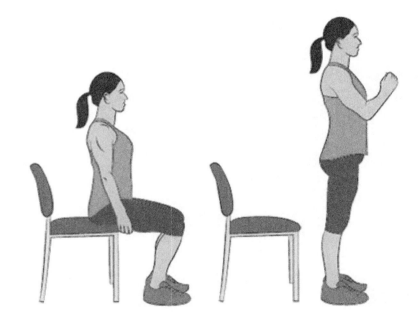

46. Chair Stands

This exercise helps in increasing your leg strength with major focus on your ankles and feet. By doing this, the chair stand movement also improves your balance, standing stamina as well as body posture.

- Other Targeted Areas: Back, abs and thighs.
- Length of workout: 6 mins
- Time duration for resting periods: 20 -30 secs in-between each set.
- Estimated calories burnt: 19 calories.

Instructions

- Sit toward the middle or edge of an armless sturdy chair.
- Then slightly lean back so that you are in a half-reclining position, with your back and shoulders straight, knees bent, and feet flat on the floor.
- Now using your hands as little as possible, bring your back forward so that you are now sitting in an upright position.
- Keeping your back straight and drawing in your abdominal muscles, slowly stand up, using your hands as little as possible again. You should take at least 3 seconds to stand up.
- Make sure that as you bend slightly forward to stand up, your back and shoulders remain straight.
- When you have fully stood in a upright position, take another 3 seconds to sit back down. That's one rep.
- Complete 2 sets of 8 to 15 reps, taking rest when necessary.

Level up: As you become stronger, try doing this exercise without using your hands.

Precautions

- Every of your movements should be slow and steady.
- Keep back and shoulders straight throughout exercise.
- If you're finding it difficult to keep your back straight on your own, try placing pillows against the lower back of the chair first, for support.

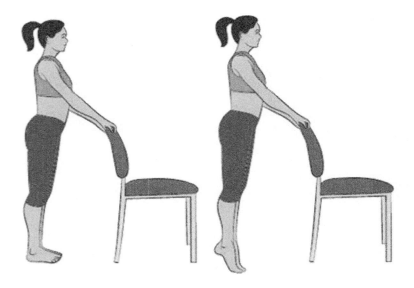

47. Toe Stand

Toe stand are another leg strengthening exercise that targets your toes and the muscles in the front of your legs. It also helps you strengthen your balance and flexibility abilities.

- Other targeted areas: Leg muscles,
- Length of workout: 7 mins
- Time duration for resting periods: 10 – 20 secs in-between each set.
- Estimated calorie burn: 19 calories

Instructions

- Start seated with your back straight and both feet firmly planted on the ground.
- Slowly, lift your toes off the floor as high as you can. You should feel the stretch in your toe as you hold that position for 3-5 seconds.
- Then lower your toes back down to the floor. Do 3 sets of 10 reps.

Level up: Perform the same number of reps while standing. You might want to consider using a sturdy chair for support at first. Then go-ahead to try standing on your own.

Precautions

- Of course, you should feel a stretch in your toes during these movements. However, do not confuse that with pain. The moment you start to feel pain, take a break!
- Do not arch your back.

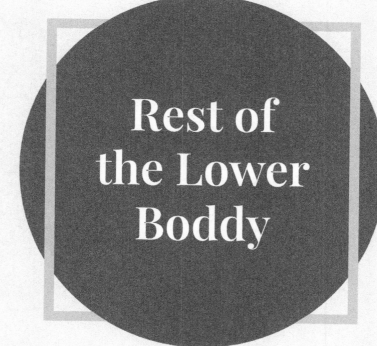

Rest of
the Lower
Boddy

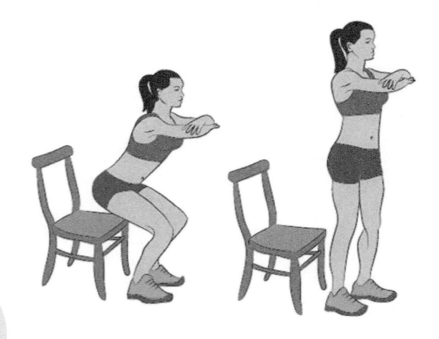

48. Chair Squat

The chair squat saves you from the intense stress of the standard squat movement and at the same time, it ensures that you don't miss out on any benefit. With the safety of a sturdy chair, you get to strengthen and stabilize your leg muscles without the fear of falling.

- Other targeted areas: Hamstrings, quadriceps, and glutes.
- Length of workout: 6 mins
- Time duration for resting periods: 20-30 secs in-between sets.
- Estimated calorie burn: 31 calories

Instructions

- Stand straight in front of a chair with your arms extended out in front of you for balance.
- Now keep your core tight as you slowly sit down onto the chair. Your buttocks should be the first to hit the chair.
- Return to the starting position by standing back up and stretching your arms out again for balance.
- Keep your back nice and straight during the entire movement. Also ensure that you breathe properly, inhaling as you come up and exhaling as you sit down.
- Repeat 10 times before resting and then going for 2 more sets.

Level up: Replace your empty extended hands with dumbbells that are fit for your strength level.

Precautions

- A recliner or a bar stool height chair is a total No-No!.
- Use a sturdy chair that is the proper height for you.
- Pay close attention to your form and make sure you are doing it right. This will help minimize stress on your back.

Rest of the Lower Body

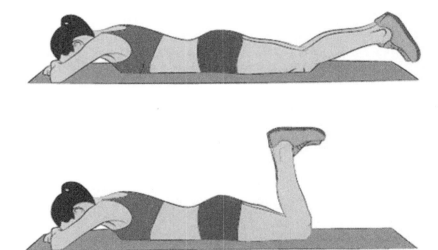

49. Hamstring Curls

Being able to balance your hamstrings, which are the muscles located on the back of the thighs, is essential for walking and standing abilities. However, aging has the potential of taking that ability from you. Fortunately, the hamstring curl is another effective exercise that will improve the balance, flexibility, and range of motion of your hamstrings. This will in turn decrease your likelihood of falls and risks of injury in that area.

- Other targeted areas: upper and lower back muscles.
- Length of workout: 10 mins
- Time duration for resting periods: 40 secs – 1 minute in-between each set.
- Estimated calorie burn: 35 calories

Instructions

- Get seated in a chair with your feet flat on the ground.
- Slowly, extend your left leg up slightly and position your left heel on the floor.
- Now lean forward at the hips and reach toward your left toes.
- Hold the stretch for 10 – 20 secs. No doubt, you will surely feel a stretch in your hamstrings.
- Sit back up and return your leg and arm to the starting position.
- Repeat 10 times before switching to your right leg and doing the same amount of reps.
- Relax a little and then go for one more set of 10 reps on each leg
- Level up: If you are sure and ready to take this exercise a notch up, try doing the same movement while standing up straight. The only difference here is that you will be bending forward at the waist and reaching towards your toes.

Precautions

- Stop immediately if you experience any pain or extreme discomfort. The best thing to do is to either readjust your position, reduce your range of motion or take a break until the pain subsides.

Rest of the Lower Body

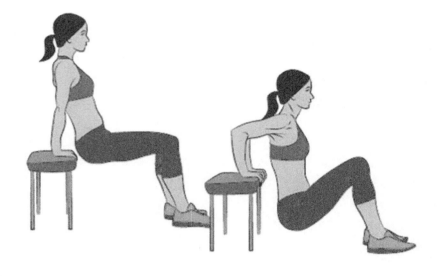

50. The Chair Dip

Chair dips are strength-training exercises that are not just simple and effective, but also very easy to incorporate into your routine. Basically, this exercise targets the muscles on the back of the upper arms as well as your lower body.

- Other targeted areas: Triceps.
- Length of workout: 7 mins
- Time duration for resting periods: 30 – 40 secs in-between each set
- Estimated calorie burn: 32 calories

Instructions

- Sit on your chair with your arms on its armrests and your feet flat on the floor, hip-distance apart.
- Your fingers should grip the arms of the chair as you move your torso forward off the chair with your arms fully extended and your knees slightly bent.
- Breathe in as you slowly lower your body back to the seat, hinging at your elbows until they form a 90-degree angle.
- Exhale as you push up back to your starting position with your arms fully extended.
- Complete 3 sets of 5-10 reps. As you build Strength, you may work your way up to doing more repetitions or sets of the exercise.

Level up: To increase the difficulty of this exercise, completely straighten your legs as you lift your torso. Also, try placing just your heels on the floor instead of the whole foot.

Precautions

- Resist the constant temptation to shrug your shoulders during movement. Try to keep them neutral with your neck in a relaxed position.

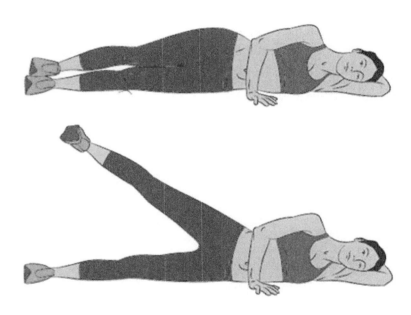

51. Side Leg Raise

Performing side leg raises is an easy and effective way to increase your lower body strength while improving its balance and flexibility abilities simultaneously. Over time, you get to enjoy your increased functional independence with reduced falls and lower injury risks.

- Other targeted areas: lower back muscles, pelvis, quadriceps, and hip flexor.
- Length of workout: 6 mins
- Time duration for resting periods: 10 – 20 secs in-between each set
- Estimated calorie burn: 36 calories.

Instructions

- Stand directly behind or beside the chair with your back straight and your feet flat to the floor slightly apart.
- Hold onto the back of the chair and take a deep breath.
- Now as you exhale, slowly lift your right leg off the floor and extend it out to the side. It doesn't matter if it is just 2 or 3 inches. Be sure that it will get better with time.
- Keep your two legs straight as inhale and hold this pose for 5-10 seconds.
- Breathe out as you slowly return to your starting position.
- Repeat 8 times on the right side then switch to the other leg and do the same. That's one set
- Perform 2 more sets.

Level up: Try letting go of the chair or using a comfortable resistance band around your thighs to make this exercise more challenging.

Precautions

- Do not lift your leg too high off the ground

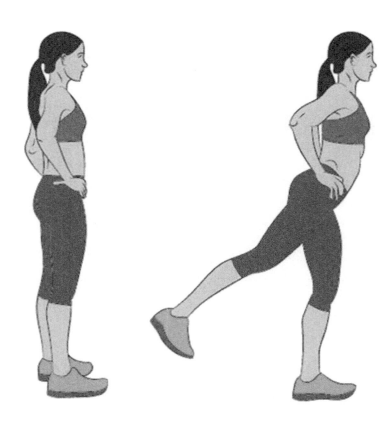

52. Back Leg Raise

This relatively easy-to-perform exercise plays a large role in strengthening your leg and lower body as well as improving your body mobility and balance. Just like the side raises, the back leg raises may require you to have some balance and Strength. So, don't be discouraged if it takes some time to work up to a perfect back leg raise!

- Other targeted areas: lower back muscles and glutes
- Length of workout: 5 mins
- Time duration for resting periods: 10 – 20 secs in-between each set.
- Estimated calorie burn: 25 calories.

Instructions

- Stand up straight with your feet hip-width apart and your hands resting lightly on a chair in front of you.
- Slowly lift your right leg and extend it straight out behind you. Again, it is okay if your leg is just a little bit off the ground. Just make sure you feel comfortable and safe.
- Maintain that position for a count of at least 5 and then gently lower your foot back down to the ground.
- Return your leg to its starting position and repeat with your left leg.
- Do this exercise for 3 sets of 5 reps on each leg.

Level up: Try letting go of the chair or using a comfortable resistance band around your thighs to make this exercise more challenging.

Precautions

- Try as much as possible not to bend your knees.
- Keep your shoulders back and chin up during the entire movement.
- Also, remember to do most of the lifting with your abdominal muscles, so keep your core tight!

53

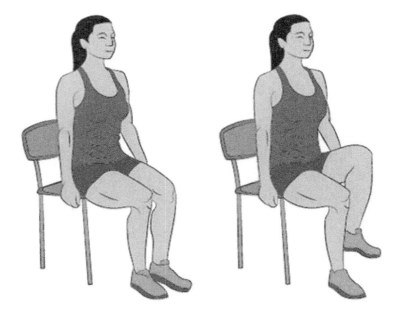

53. Seated Marching on the Spot

Though it is done in a seated position, this exercise involves you constantly moving and contracting your leg muscles which improves muscle strength, stability, and flexibility. Marching on the spot is also a great balance exercise that may help to reduce pain in your knees while making them stronger and healthier.

- Other targeted areas: Hamstrings, glutes, and hip flexors.
- Length of workout: 4 mins
- Time duration for resting periods: 20 – 39 secs in-between each set.
- Estimated calorie burn: 19 calories

Instructions

- Sit upright in a sturdy chair with your spine straight and your feet hip-width apart.
- Slowly, lift your right knee as high as comfortable then gently lower it. Also, lift the left leg and lower it.
- Lift and lower your legs 10 times, then rest and go for 2 more sets.
- Level up: Do this movement while standing.

Precautions

- Don't raise your knee too high

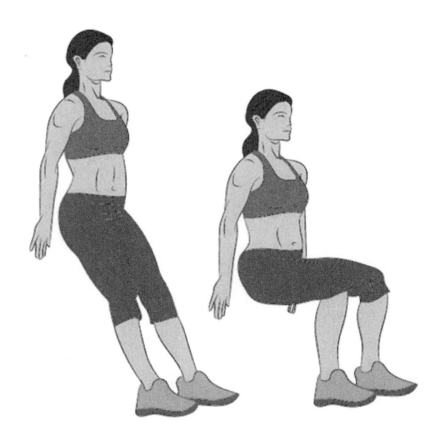

54. Wall Slides

Wall slides are excellent exercises that can help increase the Strength of your major leg muscles with an immense focus on your quads, glutes, and calves. As an elderly person, you can also use the wall slide movement to beat back bad posture and increase your body mobility.

- Other targeted areas: shoulder, neck, and back muscles
- Length of workout: 5 mins
- Time duration for resting periods: 30 -40 secs in-between each set.
- Estimated calorie burn: 31 calories

Instructions

- Begin by standing upright with your back against a wall and your feet shoulder-width apart.
- Still pressing your back and shoulder blades into the wall, bring your arms up.
- The backs of your hands should be against the wall with your thumbs at about the height of your head. The line of your upper arm, from your elbow to shoulder, should also be parallel to the floor.
- Inhale, as you slowly bend your knees and slide your back down the wall until your knees are bent at a 45-degree angle. At the same time, straighten your elbows until your arms are extended straight up over your head. However, still, place it against the wall.
- Hold this position for 5 seconds.
- Exhale as you straighten your knees to slide back up the wall until you are fully standing upright with your knees straight and elbows bent back to their starting position.
- Do 2-3 sets of 5 reps.

Level up: Add dumbbells to the wall slides workout routine.

Precautions

- Your bent knees shouldn't go beyond a maximum of a 45-degree angle. Bending more than this will place increased strain on your knees, thus putting yourself at risk for injury.
- As you build more Strength and become familiar with this movement, it is very easy for you to lose focus. However, ensure that your movement remains smooth and slow while always checking in your form to confirm if you're doing it correctly.

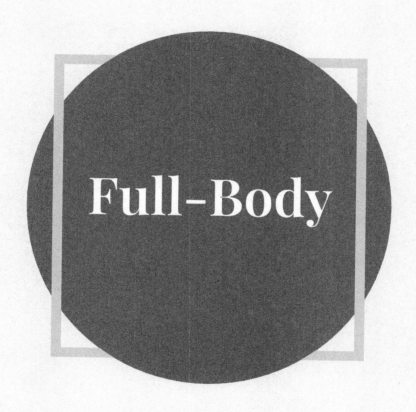

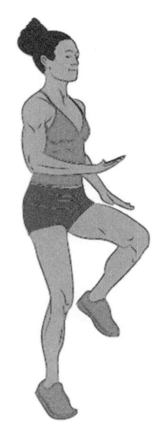
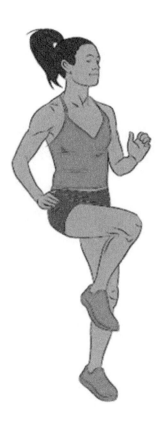

Part One: Building Muscles

55. Jog in place-warm-up

Considering the needs of an aging body, the Jog in place is an excellent warm-up exercise you can use to get your heart pumping and your body ready before going fully into the more intense strength-training workouts.

- Other targeted areas: calves, quads, and hamstrings.
- Length of workout: 8 mins
- Time duration for resting periods: 50 secs - 1 minute in-between each set
- Estimated calorie burn: 45 calories

Instructions

- Stand up and tall with your feet hip-distance apart.
- Slowly lift one foot up then the other to jog in place.
- Remember to draw in your abdominals as you jog.
- Go for 3 sets of 5 reps resting when necessary
- Level up: To accelerate your full-body strength-training from this exercise, try holding weights that are befitting for your fitness level. Doing this will also help you work your upper body as well.

Precautions

- In case this movement is too much for you, then go for the low-impact movement where you just march with high knees in place.

Full-body

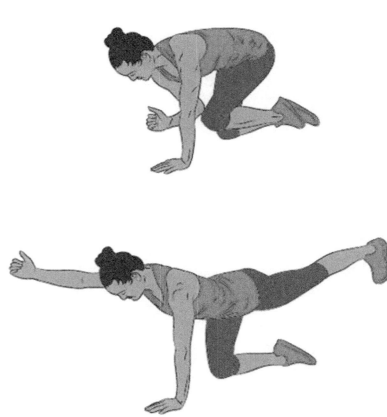

56. Bird Dog

Bird dog is a very simple bodyweight and core exercise that helps in strengthening your core, hips, and back muscles. It can also improve your posture as well as increase the range of motion of its targeted joint areas.

- Other targeted areas: Glutes
- Length of workout: 6 minutes
- Time duration for resting periods: 40 secs - 1 minute in-between each set.
- Estimated calorie burn: 41 calories

Instructions

- Get on all fours; on the mat with your hands underneath your shoulder and your knees bent at 90 degrees directly under your hips.
- Engage your core and exhale as you slowly reach your right arm long.
- While maintaining that position, extend the opposite leg long behind you.
- Hold that position for a second and then slowly lower your leg and arm back to the ground. Remember to inhale as you lower your body.
- Repeat on the left arm and your right leg.
- Perform 3 sets of 5 reps on each side.

Level up: Use a resistance band around your thighs area as you complete these exercises.

Precautions

- This exercise can seem so complicated but it really isn't complex. Just ensure that your movements are slow and steady.
- Keep your back straight!
- Avoid lifting your leg too high because it might cause your spine to curve past its natural position, leading to injury.

Full-body

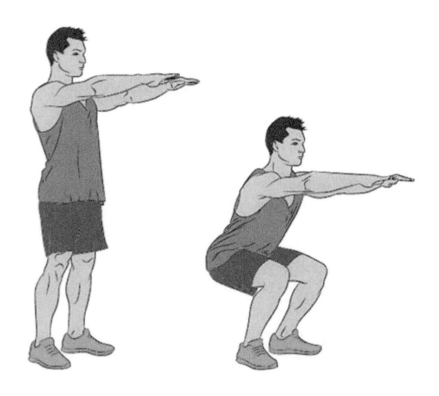

57. Sit to Stand

Sit-and-stands are one of the best legs strengthening exercises for seniors who may struggle with standing up from low chairs or from soft couches. It helps you improve leg strength, functional balance, and control. Eventually, these beneficial uses can restore your independence when it comes to your ability to get in and out of chairs and even walk!

- Other targeted areas: hip flexors, glutes.
- Length of workout: 10 minutes
- Time duration for resting periods: 1 minute in-between each set.
- Estimated calorie burn: 39 calories

Instructions

- Sit upright in a sturdy chair with your feet planted on the floor about hip-distance apart.
- With as little support from hands or arms as possible, draw in your abdominals and tip forward from your hips.
- Now, put your weight through all four corners of your feet while pushing yourself to stand.
- Once your knees and hips are fully extended, reverse the movement.
- Slowly, press your hips back and bend your knees to lower yourself back to the seated position.
- Perform 2-3 sets of 6 reps.

Level up: Try holding dumbbells as you raise and lower your body during this exercise

Precautions

- If you can't lift your body all the way to a standing position, simply shift your weight forward and lift your glutes an inch or two from the chair seat.
- Then hold that pose for a second before lowering back down. Over time, you will develop the Strength and balance necessary to rise to a standing position.

Full-body

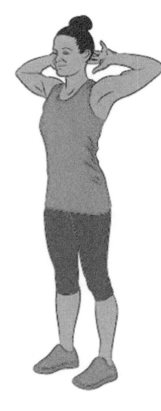
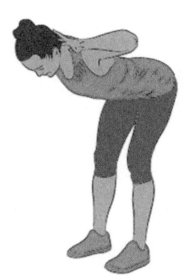

58. Good Mornings

Good mornings are great for improving your back health as a senior. It also helps in strengthening your lower-back muscles and core.

- Other targeted areas: Hamstring, abs.
- Length of workout: 7 mins
- Time duration for resting periods: 20 - 40 secs in-between each set.
- Estimated calorie burn: 32 calories

Instructions

- Stand upright with your feet shoulder-width apart and your hands placed behind your head.
- Brace your core and pull your shoulders back, as you take in a breath and hinge forwards from your hips, not your waist.
- Slightly bend your knees and keep your back flat.
- Then lean forward until you feel a slight stretch in your hamstrings. However, make sure not to go beyond horizontal. Pause a little.
- Exhale and reverse the move to stand up straight.
- Complete 2-3 sets of 6 reps, resting when necessary

Level up: To make this exercise more intense, stand on a large looped resistance band with both feet and bring the other side of the loop over your head so it rests on your shoulders. Complete the good morning exercise in this position.

Precautions

- Make sure you get the form consistently perfect right through the set before progressing to using a resistance band or barbell with plates.
- Keep the movements slow.

Full-body

Calf Raises

59

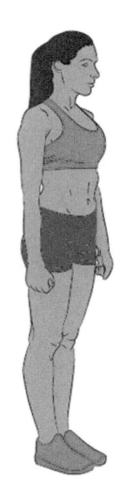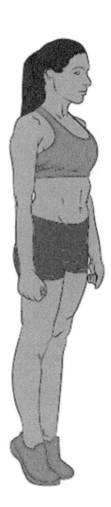

59. Calf Raises

Strengthening your calf muscles gives your lower body more power to maintain balance while executing their walking abilities. This benefit is exactly what performing calf raises can deliver to your body. They also help in pumping a great volume of blood up from your legs to your upper body and brain, so that you no longer deal with fainting or getting light-headed when standing still for long

- Other targeted areas: Toes, ankle.
- Length of workout: 5 mins
- Time duration for resting periods: 10 -20 secs in-between each set.
- Estimated calorie burn: 23 calories

Instructions

- Begin by standing upright with your feet slightly apart and your hands lightly holding onto a chair for balance and support.
- Pressing your toes, raise up on your toes as high as you comfortably can.
- Take a deep breath in and draw in your abdominals as you lift yourself.
- Hold that position for 2 -5 seconds and then return to the starting position.
- Complete 4 sets of 5 reps.

Level up: To increase the difficulty of this exercise, let go of the chair, and if that is too hard for you, use a finger or one hand to hold on with. Doing this will even help improve your balance at a faster rate.

Precautions

- Make sure your body remains still as you raise yourself up.
- If you have balance problems, keep your feet apart
- Don't forget to inhale during the upward movement phase and exhale during the downward movement phase.

Full-body

60 Bent-Over Row

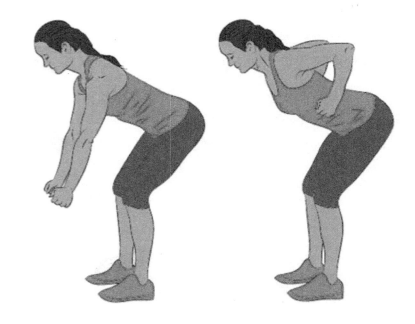

Part One: Building Muscles

60. Bent-Over Row

Bent over rows are full-body strength-training exercises that help you to improve your ability to lift and pull. By doing so, it becomes easier for you to lift a bag of sugar, empty the trash, or open up a stubborn door. These exercises basically target and strengthen your upper arm and shoulders while increasing the range of motions in those areas.

- Other targeted areas: Back and Core
- Length of workout: 6 mins
- Time duration for resting periods: 20 - 30 secs in-between each set
- Estimated calorie burn: 46 calories

Instructions

- Start by standing up tall next to a firm chair with one hand placed on it.
- Now take a step back from the chair, while slightly bending your knees, and hinging at the hips.
- Still maintaining that position, bend forward with your back straight and one arm straight by your side.
- Now bending at the elbow, pull that arm up behind your back.
- Hold for 1-3 seconds and then return to the start position.
- Repeat 5 times with that arm and then alternate arms. Go for 2-3 sets of 5 reps on each arm.

Level up: Fill up your empty hands with dumbbells that are fit for your strength level.

Precautions

- As you lift your arm up, make sure to squeeze your shoulder blades.
- Focus on getting the form right before going on to complete the reps.

Full-body

PART 2

Stability and Balance

61. Tai Chi 8-form

Originated in China a long time ago, Tai Chi is a gentle, slow, and flowing form of exercise that provides real and substantial benefits for both your body and mind as seniors.

This gentle form of exercise is excellent for improving your body flexibility, balance coordination, and strength. By doing these, loosens your tight joints and helps alleviate arthritis pains. If you're a stroke and heart attack survivor, the tai chi movement is a sure way to recover at a faster rate

Practicing the Tai Chi 8 Forms Movement gives you the essential foundational knowledge that you need to progress to the more advanced Tai Chi 24 Forms movement in terms of proper breathing, posture, balance, and concentration.

- Length of workout: 4 mins
- Estimated calorie burn: 68 calories.

Instructions

1. Commencement Pose

- Stand still with your hands by your side and your two feet together.
- Slowly lift your left foot and step sideways to the left. Make sure to lift your heel first before your toes but land on toes first.
- Move your arms to shoulder level with your palms facing down.
- While slightly bending your elbows, press your palms downwards to your abdominal level. At the same time, bend your knee slightly.

2

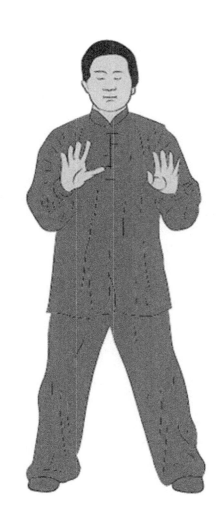

2. Reverse Reeling Forearms

- From the commencement pose, turn your body to the right corner while, dropping your palms with your fingers facing downwards.

- Now note that both arms are not fully extended. Your elbows should also be slightly bent.

- Slightly turn your chest to the right corner, stretch out both palms to the side and raise your arms upwards to shoulder level with your right hand at the rear right corner and your left hand at 12 O'clock.

- Bend your right elbow to raise your right hand, simultaneously turning your neck to look at 12 O'clock.

- Next, turn your body back to 12 O'clock and push your right hands with your palm facing forward in this same direction. As you do this, pull your left hand lower to the waist level with your palm facing upwards.

- Turn your body to the left side at the same time, dropping your left hands with fingers facing downwards.

- Turning your neck to the left side, stretch your left hand out to the side and lift it to your shoulder level. At the same time, turn your right palm to face upwards.

- Repeat the fourth and fifth steps on your left side.

3

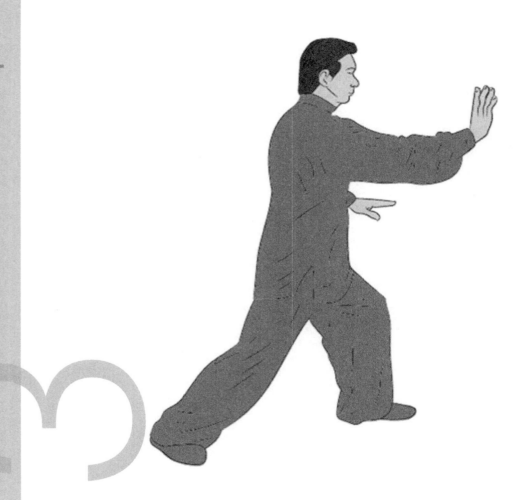

3. Brush knee push

- Still standing on your slightly bent knees, stretch out your right hand with your palm facing upwards to your shoulder level.

- Bend your left elbow and stretch your left arm across your chest with your palm facing forward. At the same time, pull your left heel in to meet your right. Raising your left heel off the ground first, lift your leg towards the side.

- As you lift, raise your right hand and lower your left arm. So, you expand the space in-between the two arms.

- Now turn your body towards the left corner, bending your left knee to 90 degrees with your right heel sliding backward.

- Push back on your right leg while turning your left palms upwards.

Tai Chi 8-form

4

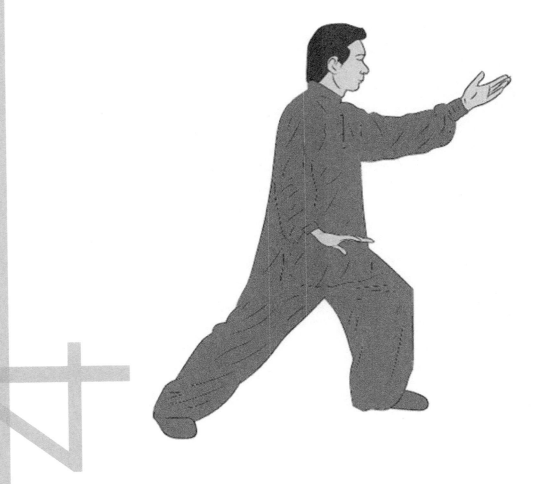

Part Two: Stability and Balance

4. Part the wild horse's mane

- Stand upright with your body facing the left corner.
- Raise your right hand to the top with your palm facing down and your left hand on the bottom with your palm facing up.
- Sit on your left knee and step your right leg towards 12 O'clock; bring your left hand lower and raise your right hand up.
- Shift backward and press your left heel into the floor, lifting your toes.
- Maintaining that pose, turn your body to the right.
- Stepping in with your left leg bringing your left hand forward too.
- Now repeat on your left side.

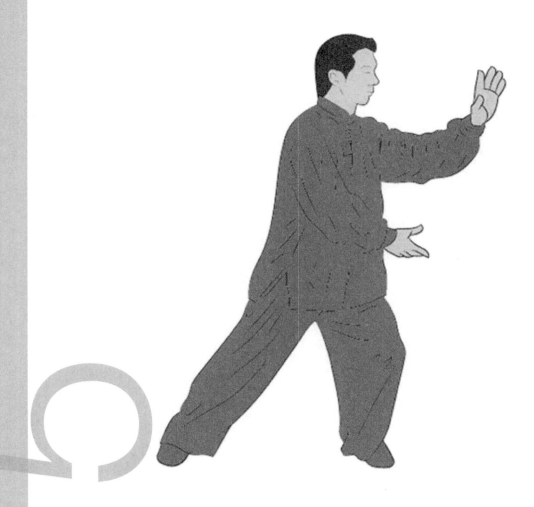

5. Wave hands like clouds

- Stand with your right hand on top and your left hand at the bottom, bending both elbows

- Extend your right leg to the side and then shift your body weight on that leg, then step in with your left leg at the same time switching your hands.

- Now shift your weight to your left leg and repeat the movement on your left side.

Tai Chi 8-form

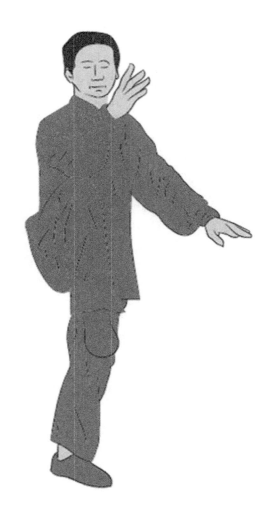

9

Part Two: Stability and Balance

6. Rooster stands on one leg

- Stand upright with your arms by your side.
- Bending your elbow, extending your left arm up. At the same time, raise your left knee to 90 degrees.
- Then lower both of them at the same time, stepping back with your left leg.
- Repeat the same with your right arm and leg.

Tai Chi 8-form

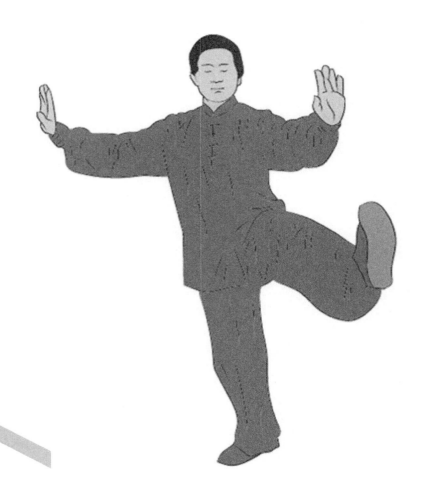

7. Kick with Heel

- Standing with your left leg in front and your right leg a step backward, extend your hands forward

- Then move back slightly and then lift your knee to 90 degrees crossing your hands across each other.

- Then expand your hands and kick your raised foot forward, lowering them to the ground.

- Switch to your other leg and repeat the movement.

Tai Chi 8-form

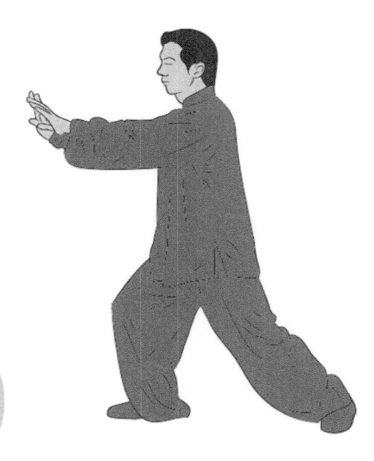

8

Part Two: Stability and Balance

8. Grasp the peacock's Tail

- Begin with your right hand on top and your left hand on the bottom.

- Then lift your right leg to the side with your right knee slightly bent forward.

- Now turn your body to the side, shifting your weight forward and extending your two hands to grasp the imaginary peacock's tail, and pulling it back to the other side.

- Then release and gently free the bird with a push.

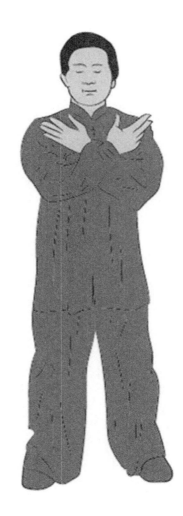

9. Cross Hands

- Stand and step your right leg to the side.
- Place both hands above your hands with palms facing outwards; the distance between your hands should be the width of your head.
- Slowly relax your shoulders and elbows as you lower your hands to drawing a circle as you go.
- Bring your right leg to the center to make it shoulder-length apart with your left leg.
- Bring both hands in your front of your shoulder's palms facing downwards and cross them.

Precautions

- Make sure that every movement is slow and controlled.

62. Tai Chi 24-form

Now that we have understood the basics, here are the more advanced but simplified 24 Tai Chi forms. They offer the same benefits as the other 8 postures we previously discussed but in a broader range

- Length of workout: 6 minutes
- Estimated calorie burn:

Instructions

Section 1

Opening Stance / Qi Shi

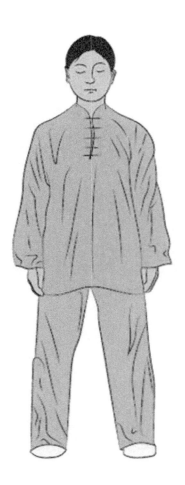

1. Opening Stance / Qi Shi

- Stand upright, feet together.
- Move you left leg sideways for balance.
- Raise both hands to your shoulder level, evenly and slowly. Then bring them down slowly.

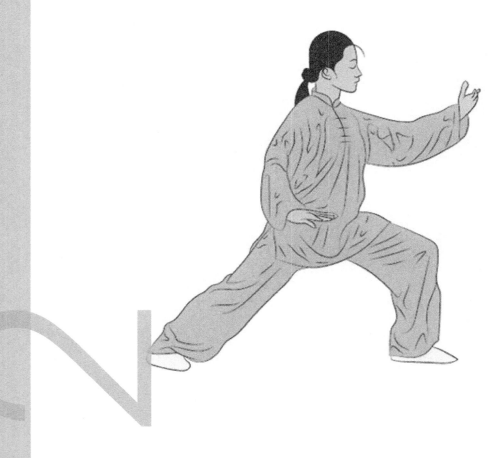

2. Part the horse mane (left & right) / Ye Ma Fen Zong

- Continuously move your weight to the right leg to form an empty step and hold a ball, take a bow.
- Raise your left hand to shoulder level and right-hand presses down to hip area.
- Rotate the left foot, form the empty step and hold a ball.
- Take a bow. Right hand goes up and left hand goes down.
- Rotate the right foot. Form an empty step and hold a ball.
- Take a bow step, left hand goes up and right hand goes done.

3

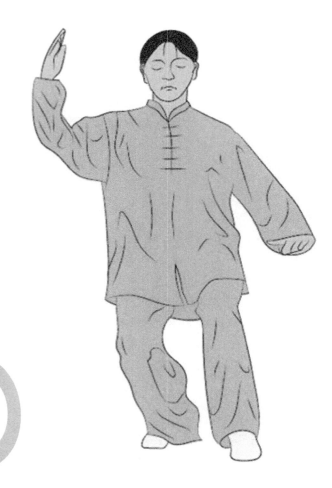

3. White crane spreads its wings / Bai He Liang Chi

- Right foot takes a step. Form an empty step and hold a ball, the right hand goes up and the left hand goes down.

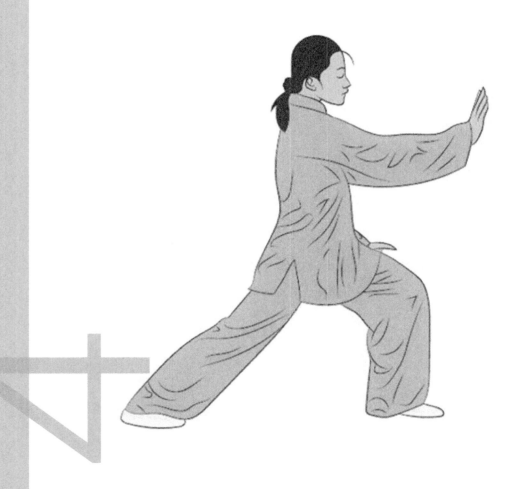

4. Brush knee, twist steps / Lou Xi Ao Bu

- Rotate the right knee. Both hands perform a semicircle movement.
- Brush left knee and push right hand forward.
- Rotate the left knee. Both hands perform a semicircle movement.
- Brush right knee and push left hand forward.
- Rotate to the left knee. Both hands perform a semicircle movement.
- Brush left knee and push right hand forward.

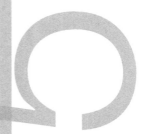

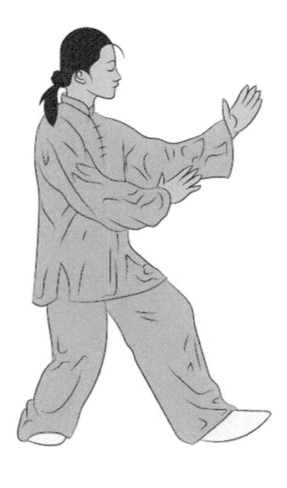

5. Strum the lute / Shou Hui Pi Ba

- Right foot takes a step, raise hands and lean on the heel.

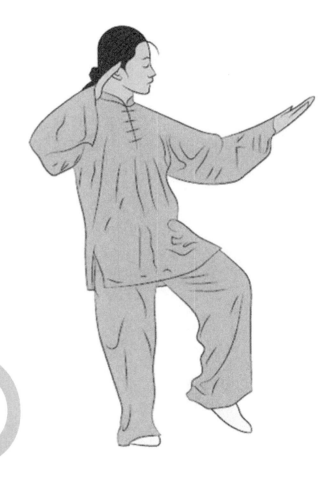

Part Two: Stability and Balance

Section 2

6. Repulse the monkey (left & right) / Dao Zhuang Gong

- Left foot, step back, right hand rotates, moves up and then pushes forward.
- Right foot steps back, left hand rotates, moves up and then push forward.
- Step back and roll hands again. Take a step back again and roll hands.
- Rotate to the foot. Form an empty step and hold a ball.

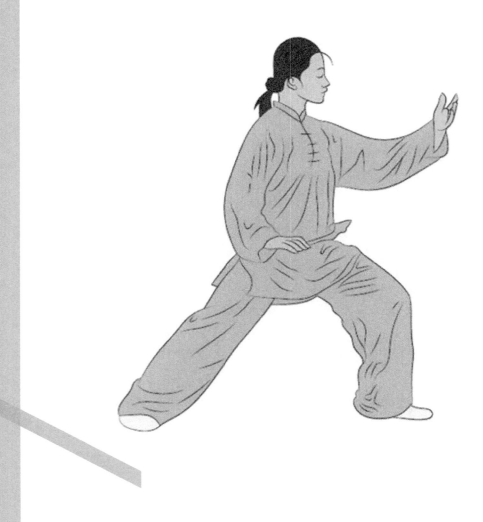

Part Two: Stability and Balance

7. Grasp the peacock's tail (left) / Zuo Lan Que Wei

- Take a bow-like step. Deflect. Push.
- Pull in. Press.
- Rotate the left heel form, empty step and hold a ball.

88

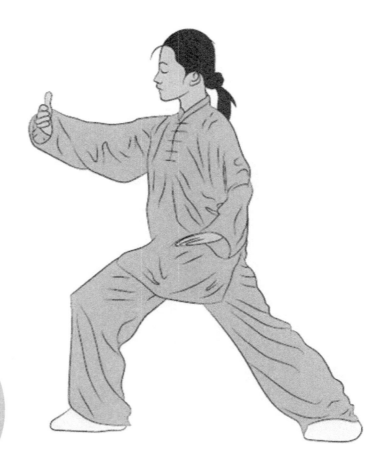

8. Grasp the peacock's tail (right) / You Lan Que Wei

- Take a bold step and ward off. Deflect. Push. Pull in. Press.

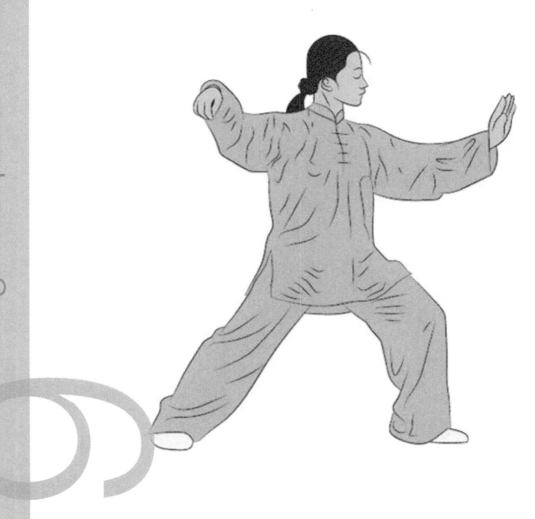

9. Single whip / Dan Bian

- Rotate both arms. Right hand bunches a hook, then forms an empty step.
- Take a left step, rotate and push left hand lean on left foot and grind right foot.

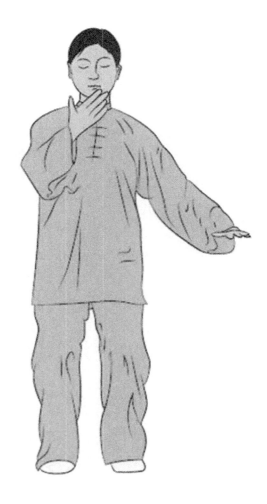

Section 3

10. Waving hands like clouds / Yun Shou

- Rotate the left heel, move the right foot to the left and wave hands to the left.
- Left foot takes a lateral step. Wave hands to the right.
- Wave hands like clouds twice again.

11

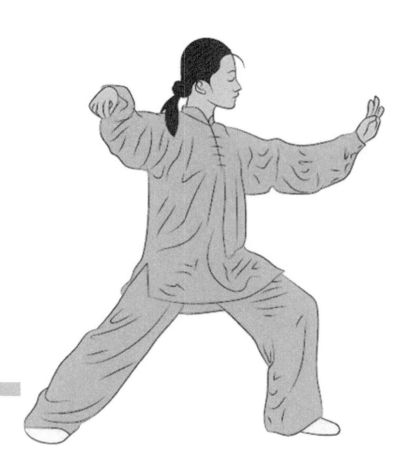

Part Two: Stability and Balance

11. Single whip / Dan Bian

- Bunch a hook and form an empty step.
- Take a left step, rotate and push left hand and lean left foot and grind right foot.

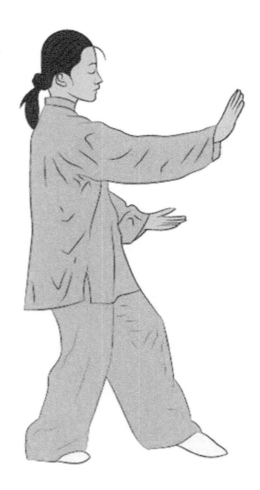

12. High pat the horse / Gao Tan Ma

- Right foot takes a step and forms an empty step.
- Right palm moves forward.
- Take a left bow step and then form an empty step.

13

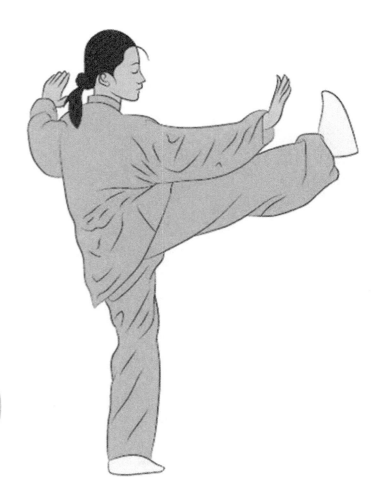

Part Two: Stability and Balance

13. Right heel kick / You Deng Jiao

- Cross hands in front of the chest, raise the right knee and then kick with right heel.
- Palm separate and move outward.

14

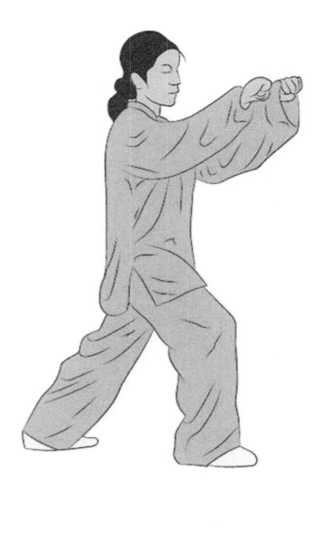

Part Two: Stability and Balance

14. Double Punch to the Ears / Shuang Feng Guan

- Drop the right foot; draw both palms back
- Take a bold step, and change your palm into fists and strike on the opponent.

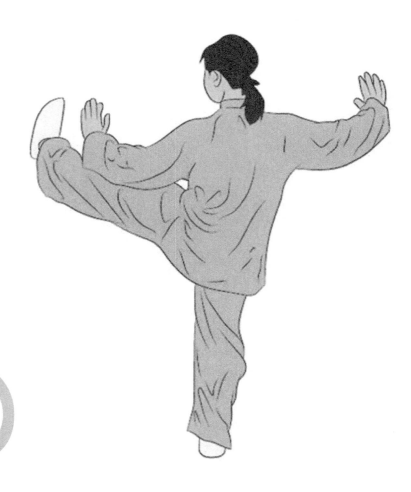

15. Turn round and left heel kick / Zhuang Shen Zuo Deng Jiao

- Rotate the right heel and form the empty step while crossing hands.
- Raise the left knee and then kick with the left heel. Palm separate and move outward.
- Left leg pulls in, left hand moves to the right axilla.

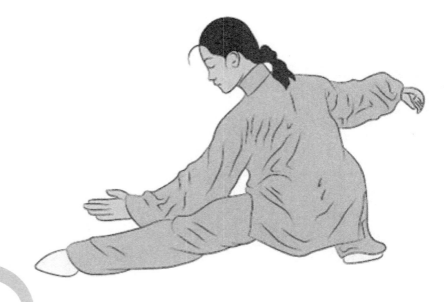

16

Creep down and golden cock stand on one leg
(left) / Zuo Xia Shi Du Li

Section 4

16. Creep down and golden cock stand on one leg (left) / Zuo Xia Shi Du Li

- Take a crouch step. Left hand threads from chest to abdomen along the inside of the leg; stand on the left leg.
- Right hand goes up. Left hand goes down.

17

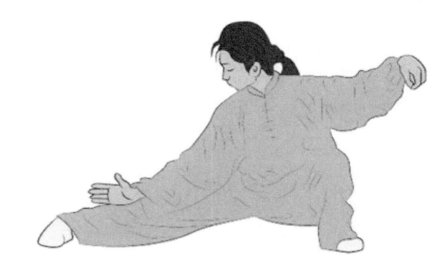

17. Creep down and golden cock stand on one leg (right) / You Xia Shi Du Li

- Land on the right toe. Rotate the left heel, right hand moves to the left axilla.
- Right leg takes a crouch step. Right palm front chest to abdomen along the inside of the leg.
- Stand on the right leg, left hand goes up, right hand goes down.
- Take a left step. Form empty step and hold a ball.

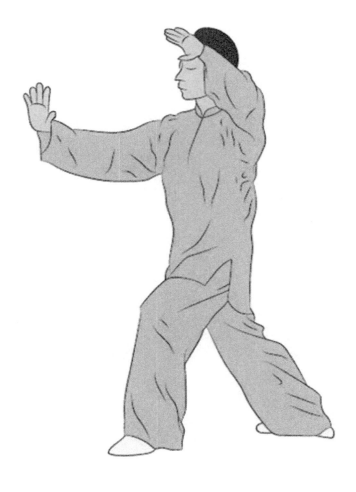

18. Fair lady works the shuttle (left & right) / Zuo You Yu Nv Chuan Shuo

- Right foot takes a bold step, right arm and rotates and blocks up, left palm pushes out.
- Rotate the right, heel form an empty step and hold a ball.
- Left foot takes a step, left arm rotates and blocks up right palm pushes out.
- Right foot takes a half step raise both hands

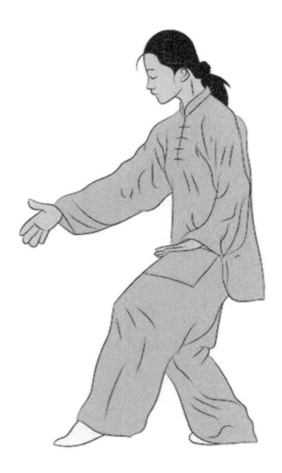

19. Needle at the bottom of the sea / Hai Di Zhen

- Brush the left knee and needle the left hand down.

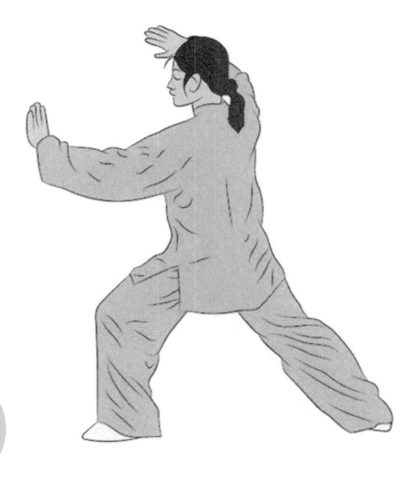

Section 5

20. Fan through back / Shan Tong Bi

- Raise hand and left foot takes a bow.
- Right hand brought up and left palm pushed forward.
- Rotate the left heel.
- Then right fist moves out and the foot takes a step forward.

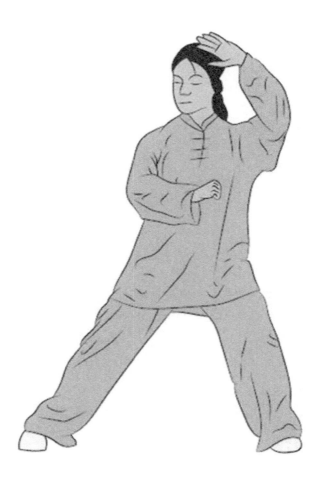

Part Two: Stability and Balance

21. Turn round block, parry and punch / Zhuang Shen Ban Lan Chui

- Left foot takes a step forward with the left-hand doing a perry and then the right fist forward.

22

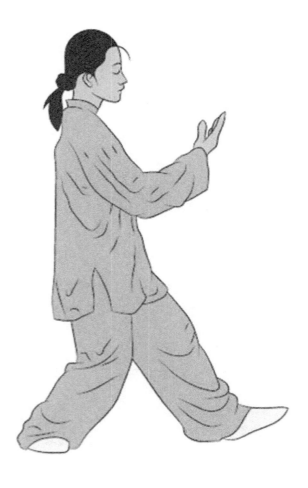

22. Apparent close up / Ru Feng Si Bi

- Both hands pull inward and downward.
- Then press both hands upward and forward.

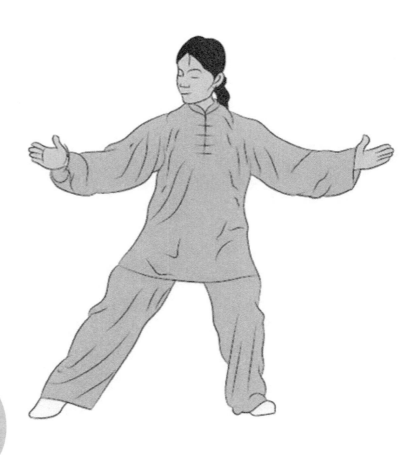

Part Two: Stability and Balance

23. Cross hand / Shi Zi Shou

- Rotate the left heel and then rotate the right.
- Open the arms and separate the hands.
- Cross the hands in front of the chest.

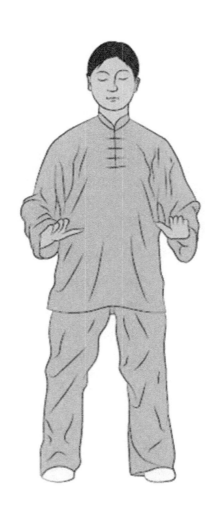

Part Two: Stability and Balance

24. Close stance / Shou Shi

- Press both hands down gently until they rest beside the hips.
- Slowly put feet together. And gently put hands along the sides.
-

Level up: You can always up to the 88 forms. Although it was condensed to the 24 forms, doing the 88 forms offers improved benefits.

Precautions

- The exercise includes a lot of rotations, be wary of this to avoid slips. Ty to perform the Tai Chi 24 forms on a not so smooth surface with flat shoes on.

Tai Chi 24-form

63

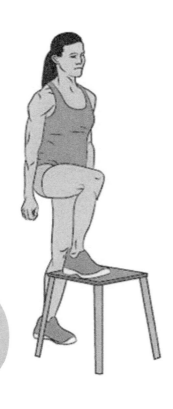
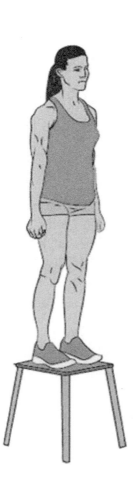

63. Step Ups

For most seniors, step-ups are the perfect exercise that comes to mind for strengthening your legs using the stairs in your home. By strengthening the muscles that support the knee, you are simultaneously improving your body balance and stability.

- Other targeted areas: hip flexors, thighs.
- Length of workout: 7 mins
- Time duration for resting periods: 30 - 40 secs in-between each set.
- Estimated calorie burn: 51 calories

Instructions

- You can perform this exercise either on a staircase with rails or on a workout step/raised platform if you have one.
- Start by standing upright at the bottom step, then step up with your right foot. Now, slowly bring your left foot up onto the stair next to your right and pause a bit.
- Step your left foot back down on the floor. You can hold onto a rail if you need to.
- Make sure that your right foot remains on the step the entire time as you step up and down with your left foot.
- Do 10 reps on that foot and then switch legs. This time, you will be keeping your left foot on the step as you step up with the right leg.
- Do 3 sets of 10 reps on each leg.

Level up: If you're holding onto the rails of your staircase, then try letting go of it to make the exercise more intense and improve your balance at the same time.

Precautions

- If you're struggling with severe knee problems or this exercise is too painful, it is highly recommended that you skip it.

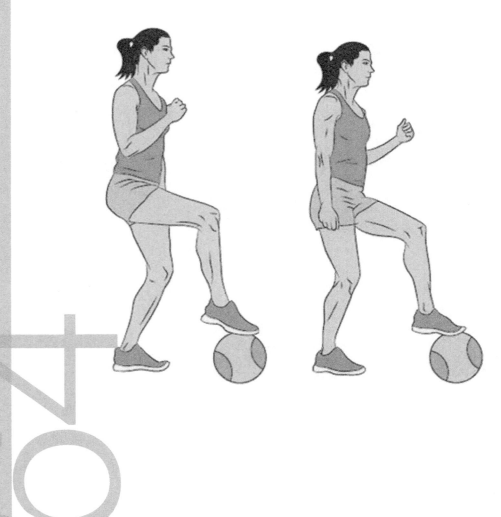

64. Ball Tap

Ball tap is another effective move that is great for the core as well as for balance and stability. Basically, it involves the use of any kind of small ball. If you don't have a ball, you can improvise by using a large book.

- Other targeted areas: Back, core
- Length of workout: 7 mins
- Time duration for resting periods: 20 - 30 secs in-between each set.
- Estimated calorie burn: 23 calories

Instructions

- Sit up in a sturdy chair with your back straight. Try not to rest against the back of the chair.
- Place a ball in front of both feet.
- Keeping your abs tight, slowly lift your right foot and tap the top of the ball.
- Lower it back down to the floor. That's one rep.
- Go for 10 reps before switching sides and doing the same with your left foot.

Level up: Consider placing your hands behind your head, as you perform this exercise.

Precautions

- Though the exercise seems quite easy, you need to keep your movements slow and steady.

The Basic Bridge

05

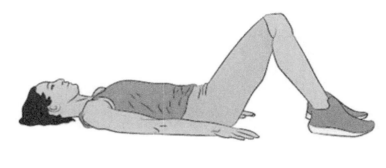

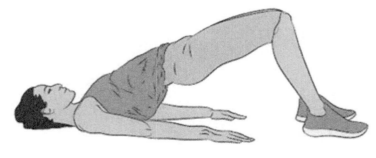

65. The Basic Bridge

The basic bridge is an effective strength-training and stability exercise that is best described as simplicity in itself. The basic bridge targets and isolates your abdominal muscles and the muscles of the lower back and hip. This, in turn, helps in improving your core and spinal stabilization.

- Other targeted areas: gluteus (butt) muscles, abs, and hamstrings
- Length of workout: 6 mins
- Time duration for resting periods: 20 - 30 secs
- Estimated calorie burn: 27 calories

Instructions

- Begin by lying down on your back with your hands at your sides, knees bent, and feet flat on the floor under your knees.
- Before you push up, tighten your abdominal and butt muscles by pushing your low back into the ground.
- Maintaining that pose, raise your hips up while squeezing your core and pulling your belly button back toward your spine. Your body should form a straight line from your knees to shoulders.
- Hold that position for 10-20 seconds, and then return to your starting position.
- Complete 2-3 sets of 5 reps, taking rest where necessary.

Level up: To increase the difficulty of this movement, you can add an exercise band, dumbbell, or exercise ball into the workout routine.

Precautions

- Avoid raising your hips too high as that can make you extend your lower back too much.
- It's okay if you can't hold the pose for up to 30 seconds. Always keep in mind that it is better to hold the correct position for a shorter time frame than to stay in an incorrect position for a longer time.

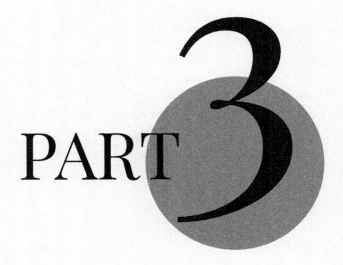

PART 3

Balance and Coordination

66. Qigong Knee Rotation Exercise

Adopted from an ancient Chinese practice, Qigong exercises are gentle low-impact exercises that are highly recommended for seniors. This particular Qigong exercise targets your knee. It not only does help to improve balance and reduce falls but also fits well into any training routine. Besides its physical benefits, this exercise promotes reduced stress, clearer thinking, and a stronger immune system.

- Other targeted areas: Hamstrings, back
- Length of workout: 4 mins
- Time duration for resting periods: 5 - 10 secs in-between each set.
- Estimated calorie burn: 23 calories

Instructions

- Stand up nice and tall with your back and shoulder relaxed; your feet shoulder-width apart.
- Bend your knees and place your hands on the knee caps
- Gently and slowly begin rotating your knees inwards 6 times then rotate outwards 6 times.
- Complete 2 sets of 12 reps.

Precautions

- Make sure your weight is evenly distributed on your legs before you start this exercise.
- If you cannot do this movement while standing, it is okay to sit.

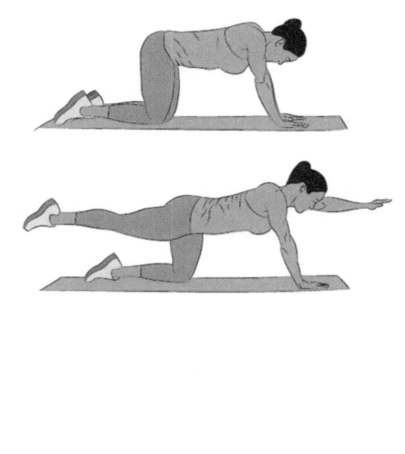

67. Quadruped Opposite Arm and Leg Balance

This exercise is another strength-training movement for seniors that improves balance and coordination in the body, most especially in your back and abdominals.

- Other targeted areas: Glutes, hamstrings, shoulders
- Length of workout: 5 mins
- Time duration for resting periods: 20 - 30 secs in-between each set.
- Estimated calorie burn: 40 calories

Instructions

- Get on all fours with your hands directly underneath your shoulders and knees under your hips.
- While keeping your back flat and drawing in your abdominals, lift your left hand to reach straight in front of your shoulder while lifting your right foot straight behind your hip.
- Now, hold for 2 - 5 seconds, and then lower your hand and foot toward the floor to return to start.
- Repeat on the opposite side with your right hand and left foot.
- Complete 3 sets of 7 reps on both sides of your body.

Level up: Use an elastic band to add more resistance around your thigh areas

Precautions

- As you extend your leg back, do not over arch your back at the top of the movement. A great way to do that is to squeeze your glutes for more stability.
- Also, ensure that your hips do not shift side to side during the exercise.

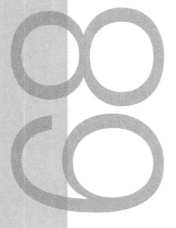

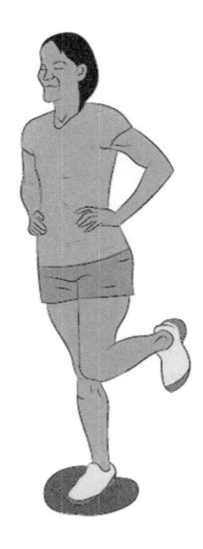

68. Rock the Boat/Balance on One Leg

As an elderly person and a daily walker, Rock the boat exercise will be quite a simple one for you. It basically focuses on improving your standing balance and coordination.

- Other targeted areas: Knee, hip flexors
- Length of workout: 6 mins
- Time duration for resting periods: 20 - 30 secs in-between each set.
- Estimated calorie burn: 32 calories

Instructions

- Stand upright with your feet hip-width apart.
- Ensure that both feet are pressed into the ground firmly, transfer your weight to your right foot and slowly lift your left leg off the ground.
- Hold that position for 5 - 30 seconds. Then slowly put your foot back onto the ground, then transfer your weight to that foot.
- With the same level of control, lift your opposite leg.
- Start by completing 2-3 sets of 8 reps per side, then work your way up to doing more repetitions.

Level up: As you work up your balance game, you can add a set of dumbbells to make it more fun but still challenging.

Precautions

- Make sure to wear your walking shoes, and stand on a yoga mat to give your feet a little extra cushion.
- If you are having a problem with balancing, you can use a chair for support.

Balance and Coordination

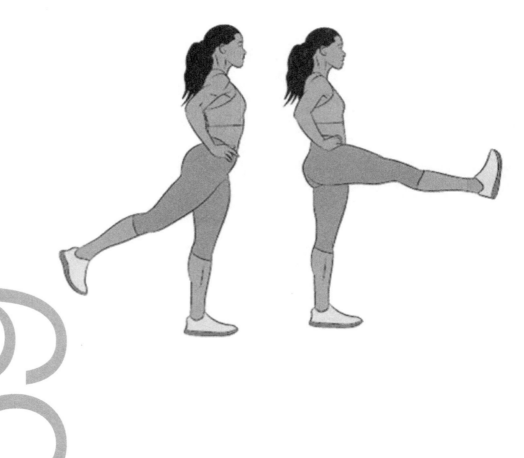

69. Leg Swings

Leg swings are another great balance and strength-training exercise that is quite effective for seniors. This exercise challenges your balance by disrupting your ability to keep your torso over your ankle.

- Other targeted areas: Hamstrings, glutes
- Length of workout: 6 mins
- Time duration for resting periods: 20 - 30 secs in between each set.
- Estimated calorie burn: 28 calories
-

Instructions

- Begin by starting upright with a chair at your side for safety.
- Now, press your left leg firmly on the floor and use it for balance as you swing your outside leg forward and backward in a smooth motion.
- As you swing, keep holding onto the chair with your ribs lifted and your head forward.
- Swing for one minute on each side before taking a break and going for 2 more rounds.

Level up: When you have worked up your balance abilities to an extent, let go of the chair and perform these movements independently.

Precautions

- Try to have a family member or personal trainer present to assist when doing these balance exercises.
- Focus on maintaining your center of gravity over your planted foot.

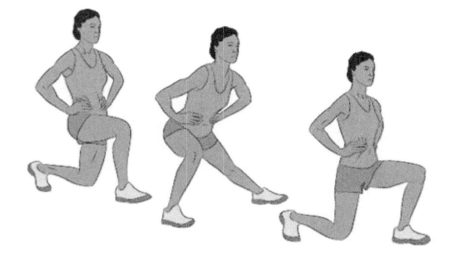

70. Around the Clock

This exercise aims to improve your static or standing balance. It helps increase the strength in your ankles and hips joints, which are vital in keeping your body stable. It also gives you the chance to expand the range of motion of your upper body. Just like the previous exercises, all you need here is to get into comfortable loose-fitting clothing and a pair of smooth bottom shoes!

- Other targeted areas: Shoulder and back.
- Length of workout: 6 mins
- Time duration for resting periods: 10 -20 secs in-between each set.
- Estimated calorie burn: 30 calories

Instructions

- Begin by standing up and holding on to a chair with your left hand.
- Envision a clock by your side with 12 in front of you and 6 behind.
- Now shift your weight onto your left leg and lift your right leg as you stretch out your right arm to the side, hitting 12 o'clock.
- Next, rotate your hands like a clock as you try to reach 3 and 6 o'clock.
- Repeat with the other side. Complete 2 sets of 6 reps on both sides.

Level up: Start by simply holding on with one finger or even let go of the chair completely. You can also add a one-pound weight to your wrist or ankle for a more challenging workout.

Precautions

- Avoid reaching too far especially if you have shoulder pain. If you cannot reach 6 o'clock, or if it is painful, stop at 3 o'clock.
- Remember to breathe normally while exercising, in through the nose and out through the mouth.

Balance and Coordination

71 One-Legged Squat

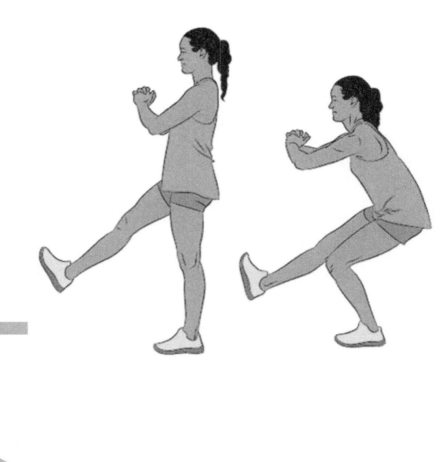

71. One-Legged Squat

As a senior, adding one-legged squats to your strength-training program is a great way to simultaneously develop strength, balance, coordination, and core stability. It also helps to tone and strengthen your legs and core muscles.

- Other targeted areas: the hips, hamstrings, quadriceps, gluteus maximus, and calves.
- Length of workout: 5 mins
- Time duration for resting periods: 10 -20 secs in-between each set.
- Estimated calorie burn: 38 calories

Instructions

- Stand upright and place a box or low chair behind you.
- Plant your right foot firmly on the ground beneath you, with the left leg slightly bent or straight out in front of you.
- Raise the non-supporting foot from the floor slightly. Slowly sink down into the squat position until your buttocks touch the box, then push back up with your supporting leg.
- Make sure to keep the knee of the supporting leg centered over the ball of the foot
- Repeat 5 times and then switch to the other leg.
- Complete 2 sets of 5 reps on each leg.

Level up: Once you are confident that you've developed your coordination, and balance enough to make this exercise more intense, switch to holding a dumbbell or kettlebell in your hands while doing it.

Precautions

- As you squat, your knee should not extend beyond your toes.
- This exercise demands that every one of your moves is slow.
- To make sure that you get the correct form, perform this exercise in front of a mirror.

Single-Leg Deadlift

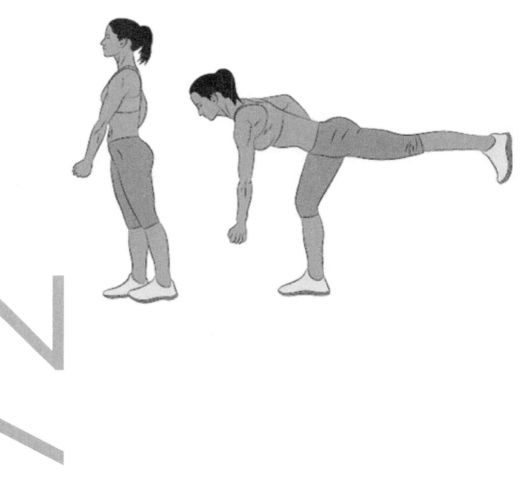

72. Single-Leg Deadlift

Performing single-leg deadlift consistently and correctly simply equals greater balance, flexibility, and stability for you even in the face of aging factors.

- Other targeted areas: Hamstrings, gluteus maximus, gluteus medius, ankles, and the core.
- Length of workout: 8 mins
- Time duration for resting periods: 30 -49 secs in-between each set.
- Estimated calorie burn: 52 calories

Instructions

- Start by standing with your right leg firmly planted on the ground beneath you and the left leg bent up behind you.
- Start hinging at your waist as you slowly bend over as you lift and stretch your left leg out behind you.
- Your right knee should be slightly bent with your arms straight. Your body should also be in a straight line from the top of your head to the bottom of your left foot
- Stop bending and pause when your torso is almost parallel to the floor.
- Slowly, rise back up and then repeat 2-3 sets of 5 reps on each leg, resting when necessary.

Level up. Add dumbbells or kettlebells to the opposite arm of the leg on the ground.

Precautions

- Keep your back neutral and avoid rounding your spine as you bend. Imagine that you have a glass of water resting on your low back when your torso becomes parallel to the floor so you must ensure that the water doesn't spill.

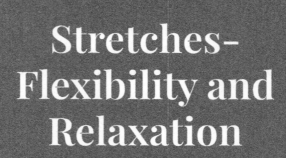

Stretches–Flexibility and Relaxation

To attain overall functional independence as you age, you cannot only focus on strength-training. Thus, just like we have discussed strength-training exercises that are great at improving balance, stability, and coordination, we will now focus on strength-training exercises that promote the mobility and flexibility of your muscles, tendons, and the connective tissue surrounding your muscles and joints.

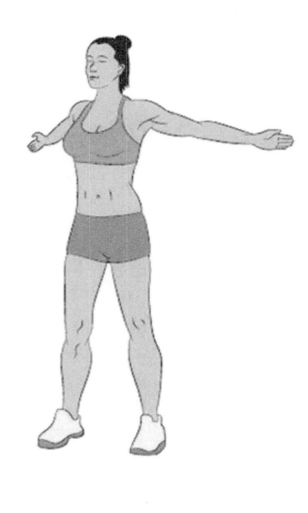

73. Chest and Arm Stretch

Poor posture while sitting or standing is quite common with elderly persons and even young ones too. Thus, it often leads to stiffness and tensions in the muscles of the chest becoming tight. The chest and arm exercise help to properly stretch and lengthen those tight muscles. Eventually, your posture will also improve.

- Other targeted areas: Shoulder, back.
- Length of workout: 4 mins
- Time duration for resting periods: 5 - 10 secs in-between each set
- Estimated calorie burn: 15 calories.

Instructions

- Start by getting seated and extending both arms to the side, palms facing forward. Inhale as you do this.
- Now, slowly reach back with your hands until you feel a stretch across your chest and front of your arms.
- Pause briefly and slowly return to the starting position. Switch to the other side. Complete 3 sets of 5 reps.

Level up: Try performing these movements while standing up.

Precautions

- Use a wall if you are finding it difficult to hold your arms up without support. All you have to do is to put your hand on a wall and step forward until you feel a gentle stretch in your chest.
- Do not overstretch.

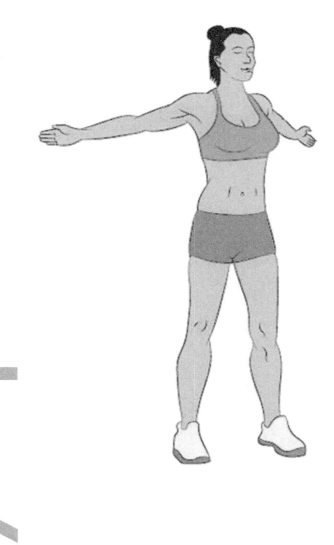

74. Hamstring/Calf Stretch

Remember that your hamstrings, which are the muscles on the back of your thigh. Thus, they are very important for your walking and standing abilities. Hamstring stretch helps relieve tension in your calves, which may cause your lower back pain and difficulty in walking.

- Other targeted areas: Upper and lower back.
- Length of workout: 4 mins
- Time duration for resting periods: 5 - 10 secs in-between each set
- Estimated calorie burn: 15 calories

Instructions

- Place your yoga mat on the floor and lie on your back.
- Extend your right leg perpendicular to your body.
- Keeping your left leg and hip stuck to the ground, grasp around the back of your thigh and slowly pull the leg towards you for 2 -5 seconds.
- Release and then lower your leg back to the ground. Repeat 5 times on your right leg before switching legs.
- Do 3 sets of 5 reps on each leg.

Level up: Try using a resistance band around your thighs.

Precautions

- Do not pull on your knee when stretching.
- Remember to inhale and exhale as you stretch.

Stretches - Flexibility and Relaxation

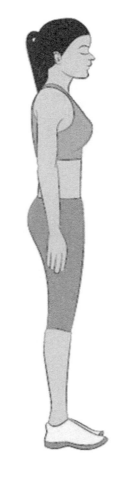
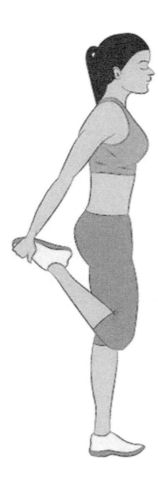

75. Quadriceps Stretch

This stretch works your quadriceps, which are large muscles on the front of the thigh. It increases your range of motion and flexibility in that area. This will ultimately improve your walking and standing stamina.

- Other targeted areas: Hamstrings, and back.
- Length of workout: 4 mins
- Time duration for resting periods: 5 - 10 secs in-between each set.
- Estimated calorie burn: 16 calories.

Instructions

- Start by lying on your side with your right knee bent and your foot behind you.
- With your hand, pull that foot towards your body until you feel a stretch.
- If you find it hard to reach your foot, you can use a belt or a towel to help.
- Repeat this 6 times before switching to your left leg.
- Completes 2-3 sets of 6 reps on each leg.
- Level up: Perform these same motions in a standing position.

Precautions

- Draw in your abdominal muscles as you pull your foot.
- Pull to the point of tension and not to the point of pain.

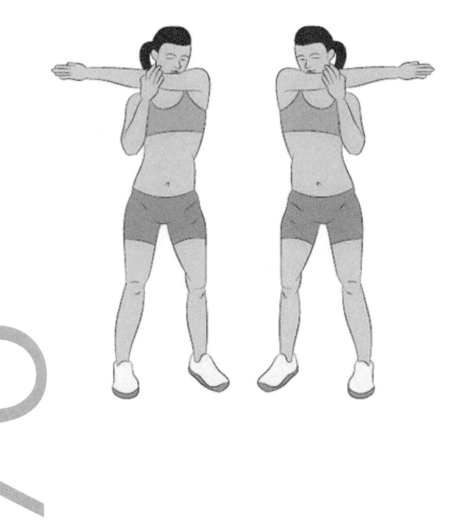

76. Neck, Upper Back and Shoulder Stretch

This exercise help improve flexibility and maintain mobility in your neck, shoulder and upper back simultaneously. By doing this, it also helps to improve your body posture and provide relief in your tight neck and shoulders.

- Other targeted areas: Core, arms.
- Length of workout: 5 mins
- Time duration for resting periods: 5 - 10 secs in-between each set.
- Estimated calorie burn: 19 calories

Instructions

- Start by standing in a comfortable standing position with your arms by your side.
- Cross your right arm straight across your chest to the opposite side.
- Then use your left arm to gently pull the outstretched right arm closer to your body.
- Hold for 5 - 10 secs and then repeat on the other side.
- Do 2-3 sets of 5 reps on both sides.

Precautions

- Never stretch your arm too much to the point of pain.

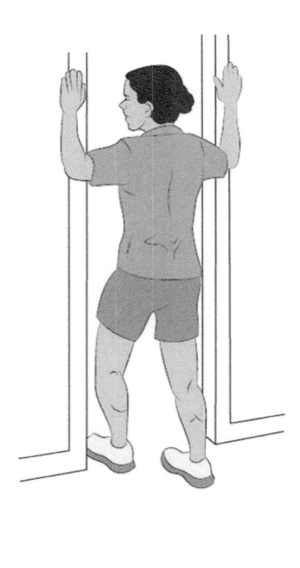

77. Standing Side Reach/Pec Stretches

This exercise offers you increased shoulder and trunk flexibility as well as a good balance. This will train your body to easily reach higher surfaces like the high shelf at home or the grocery store.

- Other targeted areas: Chest, core
- Length of workout: 4 mins
- Time duration for resting periods: 5 - 10 secs in-between each set.
- Estimated calorie burn: 15 calories.

Instructions

- Stand up and tall with your feet slightly wider than hip-width apart and knees slightly bent.
- As if you're reaching up to grab an object, reach your right hand up and out toward the same side while shifting weight to the leg of the same side,
- Maintain good balance as you reach out until you feel a stretch on the side of your trunk.
- Hold for 3 to 5 seconds, then return to the starting position and repeat it with the opposite arm.
- Do two sets of ten reps per side.

Level up: Try holding dumbbells of comfortable weights in your hands as you reach up and out.

Precautions

- Do not reach out your hands too far upwards as that will most likely put a strain on your lower back.
- Breathe normally in through your nose and out through your mouth.

78

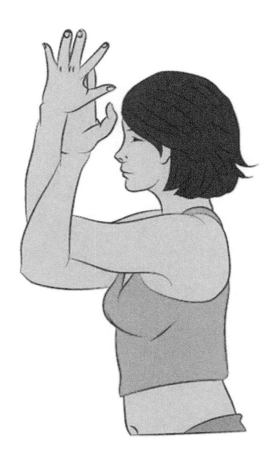

78. Shoulder and Upper Back Stretch

This movement basically focuses on increasing your shoulder and scapular range of motion. It also stretches your upper back and shoulder which in turn improves your reaching abilities.

- Other targeted areas: Chest
- Length of workout: 5 mins
- Time duration for resting periods: 10 - 20 secs in-between each set.
- Estimated calorie burn: 16 calories.

Instructions

- Sit up and comfortably in your chair.
- Then bring and bind your palms together in front of your chest, like you're about to pray.
- As you do this, take a deep breath in through your nose. Try to bring the air all the way down to your abdomen when breathing in.
- Now exhale as you bring your arms up with your palms still bound together. Straighten arms overhead with palms forward.
- Take a breath pause; then lower your arms out to the side and back to the starting position.
- Squeeze your shoulder blades as you bring your arms down.
- Complete 2-3 sets of 7 reps.

Level up: To make this exercise more intense, add one-pound wrist weights to your arms.

Precautions

- As you raise your hands, ensure that your forearms are kept together.
- Keep your chest raised and your movements slow.

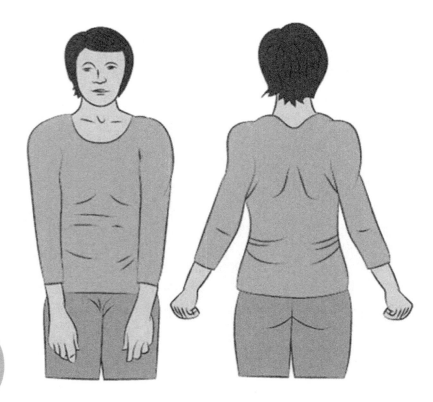

79. Shoulder Rolls

Rolling your shoulder helps find your end range motions in those joints and even expands your range of motion. By doing so, you can reduce the stiffness and tension, and at the same time improve the rate of flexibility in your shoulder joints.

- Other targeted areas: Upper back and Arms.
- Length of workout: 4 mins
- Time duration for resting periods: 10 -20 secs in-between each set.
- Estimated calorie burn: 19 calories.

Instructions

- Get seated in a comfortable position on your chair.
- Keep your core tight, as you slowly but with control, raise your shoulders upwards, then backward, and finally downwards. That's one complete rep!
- Ensure you inhale and raise the ribs as you bring the shoulders up, then exhale as you lower it back to its normal position.
- Relax and then repeat 10 times. Before taking a break and going for 2 more sets of the same number of reps

Level up: Place dumbbells in your two hands while performing this exercise.

Precautions

- Depending on its severity, take a break or totally stop if you feel pain in your shoulder joints.
- Never hold your breath.

Neck Side Stretch

80

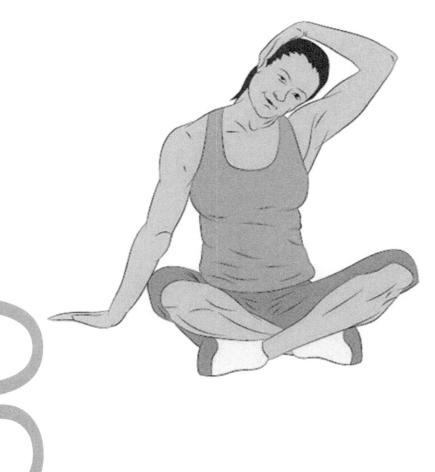

80. Neck Side Stretch

The neck side stretch helps relax the tension and stiffness in your neck by improving the range of motion in that area. This will in turn offer your relief for any neck pain.

- Other targeted areas: Upper back.
- Length of workout: 4 mins
- Time duration for resting periods: 5 - 10 secs in-between sets.
- Estimated calorie burn: 12 calories.

Instructions

- Get seated with your back straight against your chair.
- Bending your elbow, reach your right arm behind your back, and then place your left hand on top of your head.
- Now, gently tilt your head to the left. Hold for 5 seconds, then relax and repeat with the other side.
- Complete 3 sets of 5 reps on each set.

Level up: Focus on coordinating your breathing by exhaling during the stretch to relax your neck.

Precautions

- Do not hold the neck stretch for more than 5 seconds. If you have had a stroke in the past, then 2 to 3 seconds is enough.
- If you can't place your hand on top of your head, just simply but gently tilt it!
- Again, stretching should be relaxing so stop and take a break if you experience any pain.

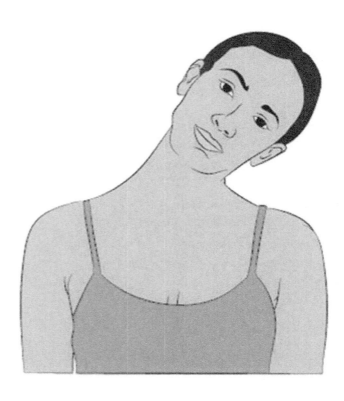

81. Neck Rotation

This exercise is an effective and safe way to relieve neck stiffness and pain, common problems of elderly people. It also helps in expanding the range of motions in your neck muscles and joints

- Other targeted areas: Shoulders.
- Length of workout: 4 mins
- Time duration for resting periods: 5 -10 seconds in-between each set
- Estimated calorie burn: 12 calories.

Instructions

- Sit upright and comfortably in your chair.
- Turn your neck to the right as far as comfortable and hold for 5 seconds.
- Then relax for a second before turning it towards the left as far as comfortable and hold for 5 seconds.
- Now, bring your right ear to your right shoulder and hold for 5 seconds. Then bring your left ear to your left shoulder and hold for 5 seconds. That's one rep.
- Complete 3 sets of 5 reps.

Level up: To increase the stretch, hold on to your chair seat when performing the side-bends.

Precautions

- Bend your neck only in the pain-free range. If you feel any dizziness when bending your neck, stop the exercise.
- Try to keep your shoulders still when turning your head.
- Make sure you are bringing your ear to your shoulder and not the other way around.

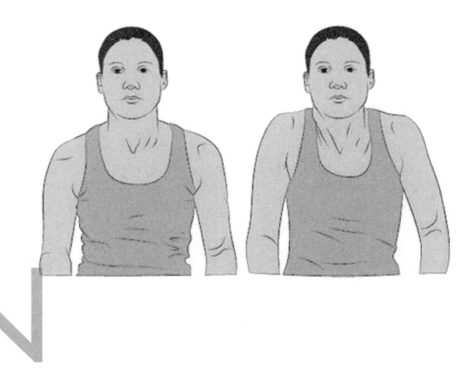

82. Shoulder Circles

Shoulder circles are dynamic stretches that gradually increase the range of motion of your shoulder joints. They also assist in keeping your rib muscles flexible.

- Other targeted areas: Arms, upper back.
- Length of workout: 4 mins
- Time duration for resting periods: 5 - 10 secs in-between each set.
- Estimated calorie burn: 15 calories.

Instructions

- Sit tall and comfortably in your chair with your elbows bent and fingertips placed on top of your shoulders.
- Keep your ribs lifted, as you slowly circle your shoulders 5 times forward and then circle 5 times backward. That's one set. Perform 2 more sets.
- To make it easier, imagine you are using the pointed end of your elbow to draw a circle on the wall.

Level up: Try doing these motions while standing up. That way, you will also be improving your balance as well as your range of motion.

Precautions

- Try to maintain your elbows high as you draw circles with your shoulders.
- Breathe normally.

83

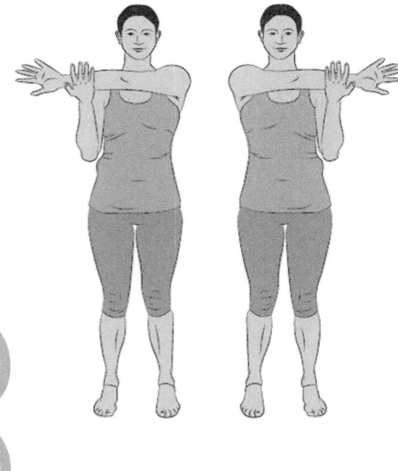

83. Shoulder Stretch

This exercise helps to stretch your shoulder, scapula, and other supporting muscles and joints in that area

- Other targeted areas: Neck, chest
- Length of workout: 4 mins
- Time duration for resting periods: 5 - 10 in-between each set
- Estimated calorie burn: 12 calories.

Instructions

- Start by sitting down with your back straight.
- Bring your right hand up onto your left shoulder and support your elbow with your left hand.
- Now, gently pull the right elbow toward your left shoulder and hold for 10 - 15 seconds. You'll definitely feel the stretch in your joints.
- Repeat the same motion with the other side. Complete 3 sets of 5 reps on both sides.
- Level up: Instead of bending it like usual, keep your elbow straight when pulling it back toward your shoulder.

Precautions

- Try to keep your elbow at shoulder height.
- Remember to lift your ribs and keep your core tight.
- Stop if there is any joint pain during the movement

Stretches - Flexibility and Relaxation

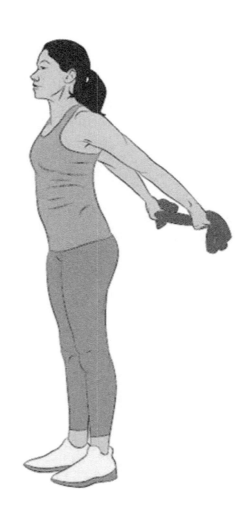

84. Chest Stretch

Performing chest stretches regularly will improve the mobility and flexibility in your upper chest and help the ventilation and functioning of your lungs. By stretching your chest muscles, you also get to maintain good rib mobility and improve your breathing.

- Other targeted areas: Shoulder muscles
- Length of workout: 4 mins
- Time duration for resting periods:5 -10 secs in-between each set.
- Estimated calorie burn: 12 calories.

Instructions

- Sit up and comfortably in your chair.
- Lift your arms and place your hands behind your head.
- Inhale as you gently bring your arms, neck, and shoulders back. At that point, you are stretching your chest and filling your lungs with air.
- Your chin should be tucked and your neck straight back.
- Now, hold that position for 1 to 3 seconds then exhale as you bring your arms down and relax. That's a rep!
- Complete 5 sets of 3 reps.

Level up: If you're up for a challenge, try leaning to the right and breathing out, while in the hands-behind-the-head position. Then in the following rep, lean to the left while breathing out.

Precautions

- Ensure that you keep your ribs lifted as you breathe in and bring the neck and shoulders back.
- Breathe deeply, all the way down to your abdomen.

085

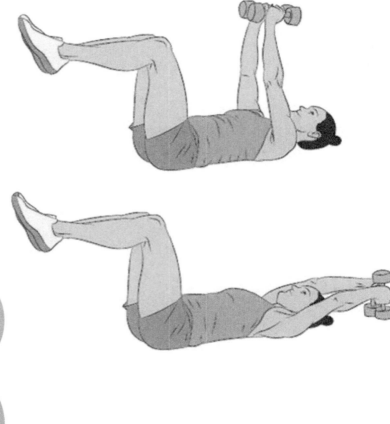

85. Overhead Reach

Overhead reach is another arm stretching exercise that strengthens your arms while giving you more range of motion and increasing your flexibility. These benefits will help you smoothly perform your daily functional movements.

- Other targeted areas: Shoulder muscles
- Length of workout: 4 mins
- Time duration for resting periods: 5 - 10 secs in-between each set.
- Estimated calorie burn: 15 calories.

Instructions

- Begin sitting comfortably in your chair with your spine straight and ribs lifted.
- Take in a deep breath as you interlace your hands on your lap.
- Now exhale as you raise your arms overhead. Pause briefly after you have fully extended your arms overhead.
- Then return to the start position and repeat 5 times. Relax and go for 2 more sets.

Level up: To make this movement a little bit more complicated, lean to the right side with your hands overhead for a few seconds before lowering them. Then repeat on the left side during the next lift. Keep alternating like that.

Precautions

- Breathe normally through the nose and out through the mouth.
- Lift your arms only as high as is comfortable. Do not overdo it!

86

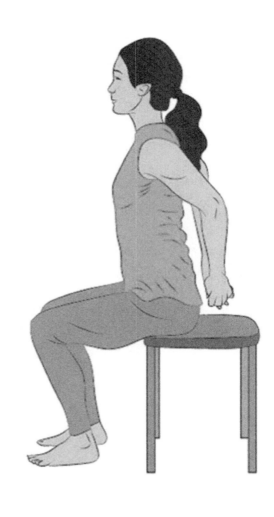

Part Three: Balance And Coordination

86. Reach Back

Like its name clearly states, the reach-back exercise improves your ability to reach behind like you are trying to reach back to hold onto an armrest before sitting down. The exercise stretches and increases the range of motion of your shoulders.

- Other targeted areas: Arms, chest.
- Length of workout: 4 mins
- Time duration for resting periods: 5 -10 secs in-between each set.
- Estimated calorie burn: 15 calories.

Instructions

- Stand upright with a chair behind you. Your back should be straight and your ribs lifted.
- Inhale as you interlace your hands behind your back.
- Breather out and gently move your arms backward.
- Pause, then return to the start position.
- Perform 3 sets of 5 reps.

Level up: Lean forward at the waist as you bring the arms back. This will force you to stretch your arms more, but be careful to not hyper-extend it.

Precautions

- Stop and take a break if you experience any pain.
- Don't move your arms too high.

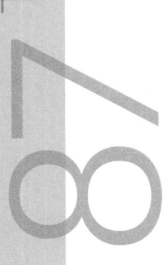

Triceps Stretch

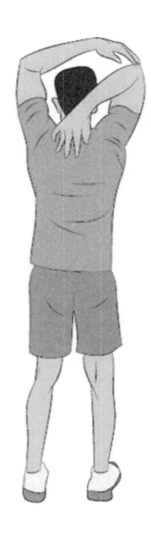

87. Triceps Stretch

Triceps stretches are great warm-up exercises that prepare your body for more intense exercises by increasing your blood circulation and delivering oxygen to muscles and the brain. Apart from this, it also stretches and improves the mobility of your triceps and shoulders.

- Other targeted areas: Chest
- Length of workout: 4 mins
- Time duration for resting periods: 5-10 secs in-between each set.
- Estimated calorie burn: 12 calories.

Instructions

- Begin by sitting in a chair while extending your left arm with your palm up.
- Tuck in your chin as you bring your left arm overhead and pat yourself on the back of your left shoulder.
- Now use your right hand to gently press your left elbow until a stretch is felt. Hold for 10 - 15 seconds. Then relax and repeat with the other arm.
- Complete 3 sets of 4 reps on each arm.

Level up: To increase the stretch, simultaneously raise your elbow higher as you try to press it with the opposite arm.

Precautions

- Keep your spine straight throughout the movements.
- Also, keep your abdominals tight.

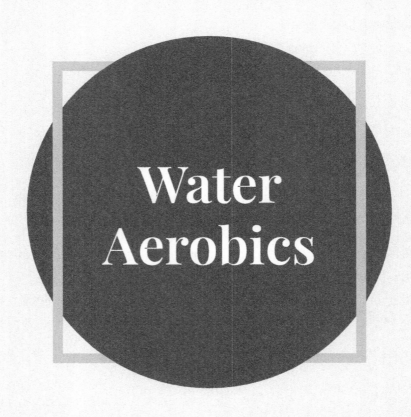

Adding water aerobics is a great way to spice up your strength training program. In fact, it can serve as a great alternative on days you don't feel like doing traditional exercise. So, start getting your swimsuits and goggles ready as we examine these four effective water aerobics you can try as a senior.

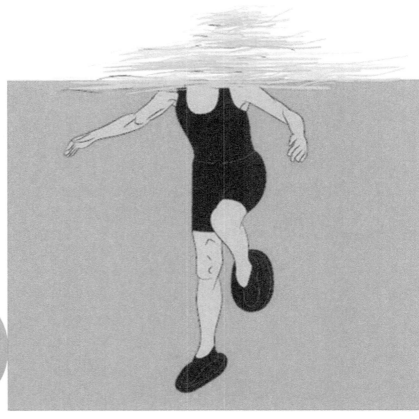

88. Aqua Jogging

Aqua jogging simply means you jog or run in water. Now, this low-impact aerobics is a great exercise to get your heart pumping and blood flowing throughout the body. It also helps in increasing flexibility and balance and, in the same way, decreasing bone and muscle loss.

- Other targeted area: Hips, knees
- Length of workout: 20 minutes
- Time duration for resting periods: 1 minute in-between each set.
- Estimated calorie burn: 230 calories.

Instructions

- Do a comfortable warm-up by the poolside for at least 3 to 5 minutes - high knees and jogging in place can work out correctly for them.
- Now rest a little, then wade into the pool until you're about waist deep. Visualize yourself jogging outdoors with your head lifted, your chin pulled-in, and your shoulder blades together and down.
- Now begin to jog to one end of the pool with your arms bent at a 90-degree angle and swinging through the water like a pendulum.
- Then jog back to the starting point again at a low intensity.
- That's 2 laps, so go ahead and perform 8 more laps. Rest a little, and then jog for 10 laps again.

Level up: To make this jogging a little more challenging, you can switch to jogging at high intensity.

Precautions

- If you are not comfortable with this jogging movement, you can walk back and forth in the pool or jog in a place using a swimming belt.
- Keep swinging your arms, and your back should be straight throughout these movements.

Leg Lifts

89

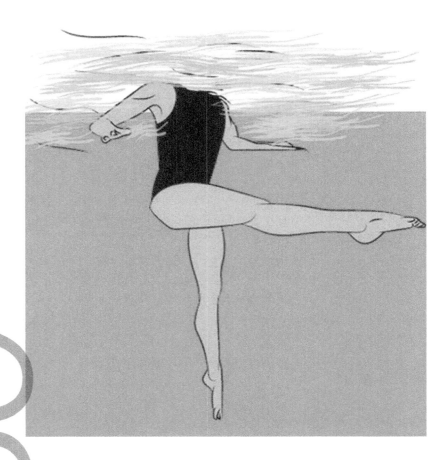

89. Leg Lifts

Taking advantage of the buoyancy and resistance of the water to perform leg lifts consistently helps to work and strengthen all of the leg muscles. This, in turn, improves your balance and cardio-vascular functions.

- Other targeted areas: Core, hip flexor and thighs.
- Length of workout: 6 mins
- Time duration for resting periods: 20 -30 secs in-between each set.
- Estimated calorie burn: 69 calories.

Instructions

- Stand in the pool and hold on to its edge.
- Now lift your right leg out to the side as far as you feel comfortable. Hold that position for 2 to 5 seconds before lowering it back down.
- Repeat 5 times before switching legs and performing the same routine on your left leg.
- Complete 2-3 sets of 5 reps on both legs.

Precautions

- If the hold feels uncomfortable or painful, lower your leg back down as soon as you lift it up.
- Avoid rushing.

Water Aerobics

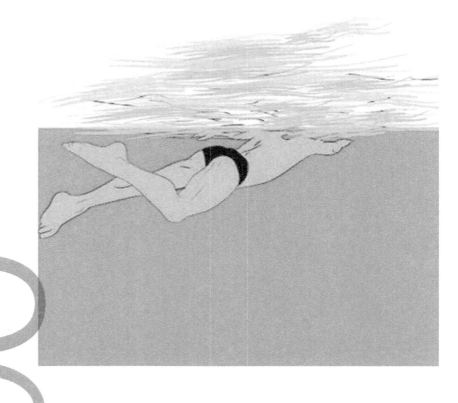

90

Flutter Kicking

90. Flutter Kicking

Flutter kicking is a great low-impact cardio exercise for seniors. It basically targets and works your abdominal muscles and lower body, increasing strength and mobility in those areas. You will need a floating device like kickboard or pool noodle to keep your upper body afloat during this exercise.

- Other Targeted Areas: hip flexor, gluteus muscles.
- Length of workout: 6 mins
- Time duration for resting periods: 20 -30 secs in-between each set.
- Estimated calories burnt: 34 calories.

Instructions

- Get into the water and hold your floating device out in front of you, with your legs hanging towards the bottom of the pool.
- Once you are comfortable, begin to scissor kick your feet front-to-back rapidly across the pool.
- Your head and upper body should be kept afloat throughout the movement.
- As you kick, point your toes and keep your legs straight as comfortable.
- Repeat this movement 12 times, taking a break and then going ahead to do one more set of 12 reps.

Level up: As you begin to feel more comfortable in the water, you can try doing the exercise without the floating device.

Precautions

- Whichever you do this movement with or without a floating device, make sure you only kick at a steady tempo that doesn't weaken you too quickly but also gets the heart pumping.

Water Aerobics

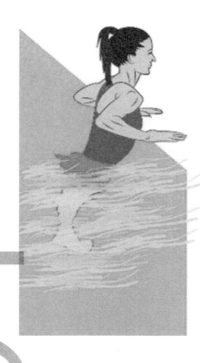
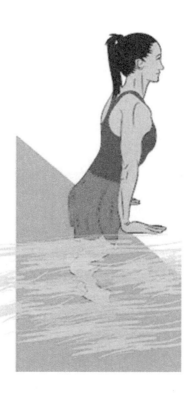

91. Standing Water Push-Ups

Often, the downside to traditional push-ups is that it involves putting too much pressure on most joints in your upper body. However, this water aerobics variation of standing push-ups cuts out those faults. It helps you increase strength and mobility in the muscles of your upper body.

- Other targeted areas: Arms, chest, shoulders.
- Length of workout: 5 mins
- Time duration for resting periods: 10 - 20 secs in between each set.
- Estimated calorie burn: 60 calories.

Instructions

- Begin by standing with your chest 2cm away from the edge of the pool and your hands a little wider than shoulder-width apart on the edge of the pool.
- Your elbows should be in line with your shoulders, and your feet shouldn't be touching the bottom of the pool.
- Inhale and slowly bend your arms as you lower yourself into the water till your elbows are bent to 90 degrees.
- Move as if you are getting out of the water and push yourself back out of the water. Exhale as you push up.
- Complete 3 sets of 4 reps, resting when necessary.

Level up: Make your upward and downward arm movement slower.

Precautions

- Be careful not to push your arms too hard mostly if you haven't figured out your limits.
- To reduce the strain on your arms during the push-ups, you can add a small jump.
- Keep your shoulders down, and avoid locking your elbows.

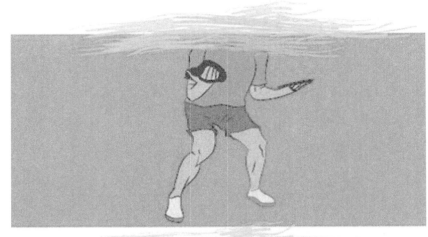

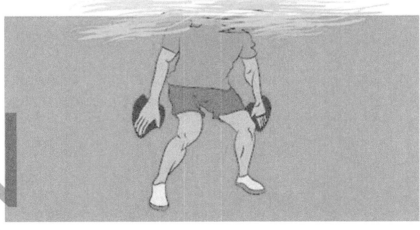

92. Arm Curls

The technique of this arm curl exercise still remains the same as the traditional one. However, the resistance of the water will work your muscles harder as you move them up and down. To perform this exercise, you will be needing a pair of dumbbells!

· Other targeted areas: Triceps, shoulders, chest.
· Length of workout: 5 mins
· Time duration for resting periods: 5 secs in-between each set.
· Estimated calorie burn: 60 calories.

Instructions

· Stand in the middle of the pool with the water dumbbells weights in your arms.
· Stretch those arms straight to the side, parallel to the bottom of the pool, with your palms facing downwards.
· Now, slowly push the dumbbells down as you bend your elbows together toward your armpits.
· Your shoulders should be still during this movement. Exhale as you bend.
· Pause for about 2 seconds, and then gently extend your arms back to the original position. Take in a deep breath as you extend your elbows.
· Complete 2-3 sets of 5 reps.

Level up: Switch to dumbbells of heavier weight.

Precautions

· Only from your shoulders to your lower body should be submerged in the water.
· Water weights are not mandatory. If you will be putting yourself at risk with the extra resistance, then ditch it and just repeat this exercise with you just clenching your fist.

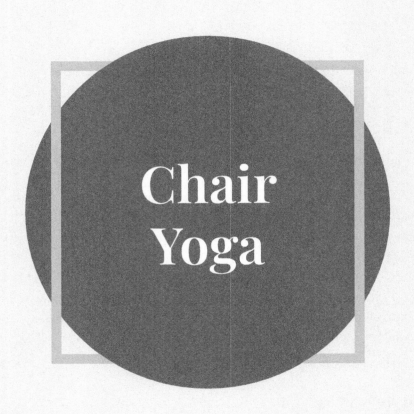

Chair
Yoga

Chair yoga is a highly beneficial low-impact form of yoga for seniors of any fitness level. All you need is an armless, stable chair and comfortable clothing that isn't too tight or baggy.

93

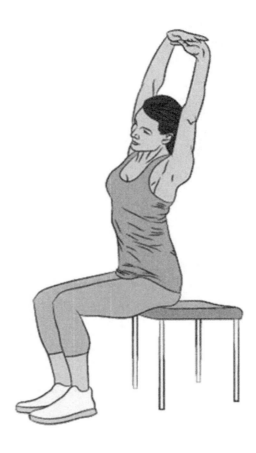

93. Overhead Stretch

These exercises basically help you relieve your joint pains and improve your flexibility, blood circulation, and balance.

- Other targeted areas: Shoulders, back.
- Length of workout: 4 mins
- Time duration for resting periods: 10 - 20 secs in-between each set.
- Estimated calorie burn: 24 calories.

Instructions

- Get seated with your front-facing forward, your back straight, and your arms down by your sides.
- Keep your core tight as you take a long, deep breath in and slowly stretch your arms upward to the ceiling. Go as high as comfortable.
- Hold this position for about 5- 20 seconds, and lower your arms back downward. Make sure you do with a long exhale.
- Do 2 sets of 8-10 reps.

Level up: If you are up for a challenge, try using dumbbells to create extra resistance.

-

Precautions

- Keep your spine neutral throughout the entire movement.
- Do not over-extend your arms.

Chair Yoga

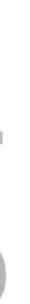
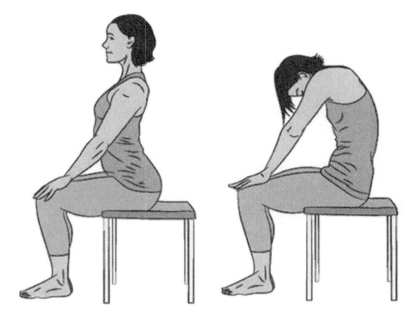

94. Seated Cow Stretches

This exercise is a yoga essential that helps ease pain in your spine and improve blood circulation in the discs in your back.

- Other targeted area: Core
- Length of workout: 5 mins
- Time duration for resting periods:
- Estimated calorie burn: 35 calories.

Instructions

- Get seated at the edge of your chair with your back as straight.
- Engage your core muscles and take in a deep breath as you gently arch your back as far as it is comfortable.
- Maintain that position for 3 to 5 breaths. Then bring your back to its original position.
- Complete 3 sets of 5 reps.

Precautions

- Remember that this exercise is supposed to be fun and comfortable, so stop when it begins to worsen.

05

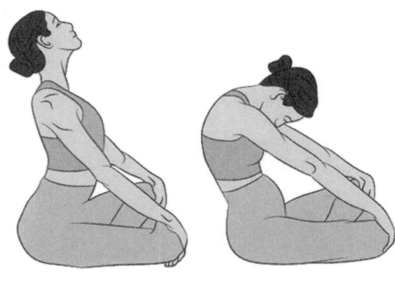

95. Seated Cat Stretches

This is the twin of the seated cow stretch movement. Often, they are combined as one. It is also useful for building a healthy spine.

- Other targeted areas: Abdominals, shoulders.
- Length of workout: 4 mins
- Time duration for resting periods: 5 secs in-between each set.
- Estimated calorie burn: 28 calories.

Instructions

- Begin by sitting on the edge of the chair with your spine in a neutral position.
- Now for the "cat" position, your shoulders should be directly above your hips as your back curves into a forward arch.
- Hold this position for 3 to 5 breaths before returning to your original seated position. That's one rep.
- Perform 3 sets of 5 reps, resting when necessary.

Level up: Deepen the intensity by drawing your navel in as firmly as possible during the pose.

Precautions

- This stretch should always be pain-free. So, if you feel any pain, gently back out.

Chair Yoga

Seated Mountain Pose

96

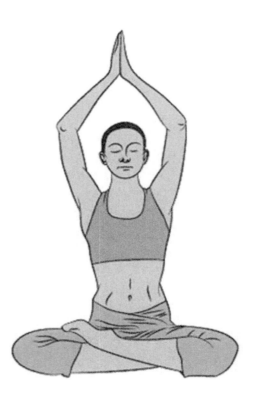

96. Seated Mountain Pose

The seated mountain pose is perfect for stretching your upper body's muscles, especially your trunk and shoulders. It helps relieve your joints of stress and strengthens them instead. As you stretch, your body is supposed to look like a mountain.

- Other targeted areas: Waist, hamstrings.
- Length of workout: 8 mins.
- Time duration for resting periods: 30-40 secs in-between each set.
- Estimated calorie burn: 56 calories

Instructions

- Sit comfortably in a sturdy chair with your back straight.
- Stretch your hands forward and interlock the fingers.
- With your hands and interlocked fingers still stretched in front of you, turn your palms outward.
- Now slowly raise the hands above your head, at the same time turning your palms upwards towards the roof.
- Make sure to align your head, trunk, and hands in a straight line as your Gaze straight ahead in a relaxed way.
- Breathe normally and make sure both your upper and lower body are stable.
- Remain in this position for about 10 secs -30 secs as long as comfortable.
- To return to the original position, gently turn the palm inwards and bring down the hands. Release the interlocked fingers and let your palms rest on the thighs.
- Complete 4 sets of 3 reps

Precautions

- If you experience aching in your hands or shoulders at any position, make sure you can release the pose and take a break.
- Relax the whole upper body while keeping it straight and firm through the movement.

Chair Yoga

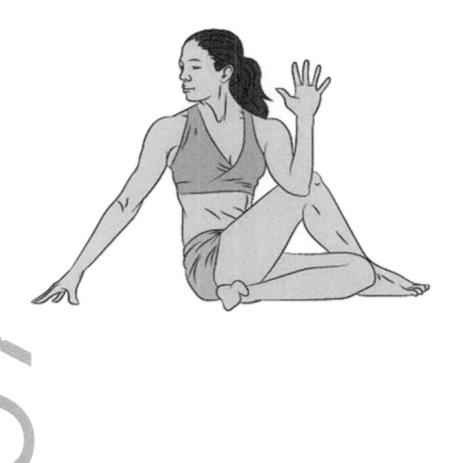

97. Seated Twist

This twisting exercise is a safe way to improve the flexibility of the spine, shoulders, and hips. It also keeps the joints in those areas very active, which indeed is a helpful necessity for seniors

- Other targeted areas: Neck, upper back, and arms.
- Length of workout: 4 mins
- Time duration for resting periods: 10 - 20 secs in-between each set.
- Estimated calorie burn: 28 calories.

Instructions

- Sit sideways in your chair, with your knees over the chair's right side and the back of the chair next to your right arm.
- Your back should be straight and not rested against the chair.
- Maintaining that pose, hold the back of the chair with both hands and inhale deeply.
- Slowly turn your body toward the back of the chair while exhaling.
- Hold this position for three to five 5 breaths and then turn back to your original position with the same control level.

Precautions

- Twist your body only within the range of comfort

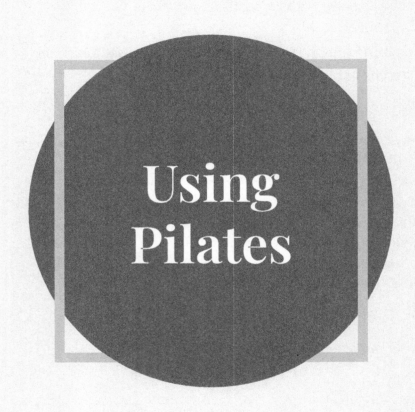

Using
Pilates

Pilates movement is a gentle strength-training exercise that has proven to be quite a useful tool for seniors looking to increase their physical strength and flexibility levels.

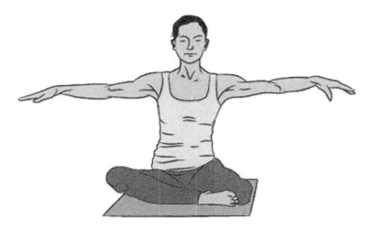

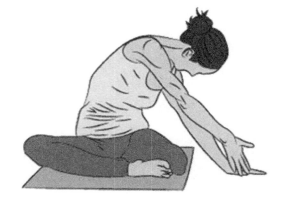

98. Mermaid Movement

This exercise is a Pilates mat exercise that lengthens your side body and provides inner body flow. It also helps in keeping the scapula muscle settled in your back.

- Other targeted areas: Obliques, shoulders, inner thighs
- Length of workout: 5 mins
- Time duration for resting periods:
- Estimated calorie burn: 20 calories.

Instructions

- Start by sitting on your mat with both of your legs folded to the left side. Make sure the back foot is flat on the floor to protect your knee.
- Also, place your right hand on the floor; this will give the body support when you sit up.
- While keeping the left shoulder down and away from your ear, extend your left arm straight up and lengthen the spine as the body stretches to the side.
- The opposite (support) hand will move farther away from the body to increase the stretch
- To return back to start, send the left sit bone down and then engage the core to bring the torso up.
- Repeat 3 times and then switch the other side to complete the full movement.
- Complete 2 sets of 3 reps on each side.

Level up: As you become more comfortable with this stretch, you may try performing an arm circle with your upper arm at the top of the stretch.

Precautions

- Do not let your ribs pop forward as you curve to the side.
- Avoid arching your back or raising your shoulders.

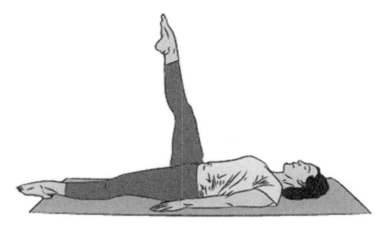

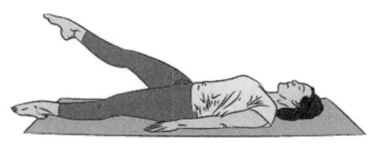

99. Leg Circle

Leg circles are classical Pilates mat exercise that is very effective for increasing your core strength and improving pelvic stability.

- Other targeted areas: Abdominal muscles, quads, hamstrings
- Length of workout: 8 mins
- Time duration for resting periods: 40- 1 minute's break in-between each set.
- Estimated calorie burn: 30 calories.

Instructions

- Lie on your back with your legs extended on the floor, arms by your sides.
- Draw in your abdominal muscles and stabilize your pelvis and shoulders.
- Now slowly pull your left knee in towards your chest and then extend it straight towards the roof.
- Cross that extended leg up and over the body, such that it angles up toward the opposite shoulder and over your right leg.
- Exhale and then lower the leg down towards the center line in a circling motion.
- Exercise control. You gently carry the open leg out to the side and then sweep it around back to center at your starting position.
- Perform two to three circles in this direction, then reverse by exhaling and then reaching your extended leg out to the side and then circling back toward and over the body.
- Stretch appropriately before switching legs. Do that by climbing your hands up your left leg to hold the ankle. Hold the position for two full breath cycles, gently pulling the leg closer and closer to you.
- Then repeat the first four steps on the opposite leg and finish with another stretch.
- Perform 2 sets of 5 reps on each leg.

Level up: Increase the size of the circle you make with your leg, and also try incorporating a resistance band into this exercise.

Precautions

- Keeping your shoulders and pelvis stable more important than making big circles with your legs.

Side Circles

100

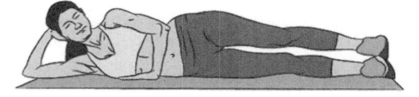

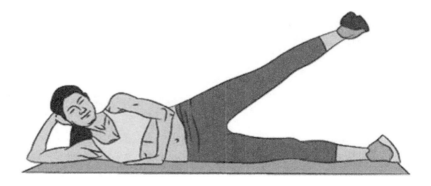

100. Side Circles

Just like the leg circles, this exercise also improves hip joint flexibility and lower body balance.

- Other targeted areas: Quadriceps, glutes.
- Length of workout: 5 mins
- Time duration for resting periods: 20 - 30 secs in-between each set.
- Estimated calorie burn: 25 calories.

Instructions

- To perform the side circle movement, lay on your left side and extend your leg towards the ceiling.
- Still maintaining that pose and engaging your core, slowly move your extended counterclockwise in small circles.
- Draw 2-3 circles and then reverse and move your leg clockwise to draw about 2-3 small circles.
- Gently lower your leg and switch to your right sides, repeating the same motions.
- Complete 2 sets of 4-6 reps on each leg.

Level up: Try increasing the size of the circle you draw with your legs. You can also add an elastic band to increase the resistance.

Precautions

- Only go as high as you feel comfortable.

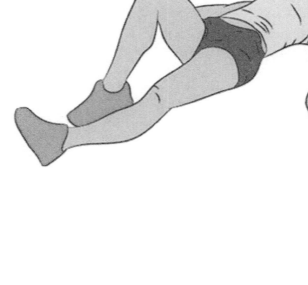

101. Foot Slides

Performing the foot slides pilates movement helps to activate and strengthen your deep core muscles and your hamstrings. By doing this, also aids in increasing your pelvic stability and balance.

- Other targeted areas: Ankle, knee.
- Length of workout: 4 mins
- Time duration for resting periods: 5 secs in-between each set
- Estimated calorie burn: 16 calories.

Instructions

- Begin by lying on your back with your knees bent and your core tight.
- Take a deep breath in and slowly slide your right foot out along the floor. Imagine that you're dragging your heel through sticky mud. That should make it easy.
- Keep the pelvis still and back relaxed throughout.
- Then exhale and slowly return to the starting position.
- Perform 3 sets of 5 reps on each leg.

Level up: You may add a 2-to-5-pound ankle weight to your leg.

Precautions

- Avoid lying on the bare floor; use a yoga mat or any comfortable mat.

90 Days Strength Training Exercise

Day 1	Day 2	Day 3	Day 4	Day 5
Triceps Stretch Biceps Curl Finger Bends Pelvic tilt	Shoulder Circles Overhead stretch Finger Lifts Dumbbell Bench Press	Step up Leg swings Knee extensions	Seated Twist Lat Pull with Band Shoulder and Upper Back Stretch	Tai Chi 8 forms Mermaid movement

Day 6	Day 7	Day 8	Day 9	Day 10
Upright Rows Wall Angels Neck rotation stretch	Wall Push-Ups Forward punches Shoulder Rolls	Lower back stretch Bent-Over Row Seated Twist Reverse Flyers	Triceps Extension Lying hip bridges Wrist Stretches Good Mornings	Chair Squat Sit to Stand Reach back Seated Marching on the spot

Day 11	Day 12	Day 13	Day 14	Day 15
Neck Side Stretch Shoulder Overhead Press Assisted Finger abductions stretch Hip Abductions	Hamstring/Calf Stretch Bird dog Qigong knee rotation Wall slides	Triceps stretch Seated Cow stretches Seated Cat stretch Ball Tap	Chest Squeeze with Med Ball Triceps extension Ball squeezes Ball Tap	Bicep curls Hand Open/Closes Bent Knee Raise Side Leg Raise Toe Raises

Day 16	Day 17	Day 18	Day 19	Day 20
Wall Angels Neck Rotation Squat Curl Knee Lift Quadriceps stretch Ankle Circles	Chest stretches Chest Squeeze with Med Ball Mid-Back Extension Hip Abductions	Finger Marching Standing Side Reach Shoulder Shrugs Overhead reach	Triceps stretch Diagonal Shoulder Raise Hip Marching Toe Raise	Reverse Flyers Wall Slides Shoulder Overhead Press Knee Thrusters

Day 21

Quadruped
Opposite Arm
and Leg Balance
Quadriceps
Stretch
Leg circles

Day 22

Rock the boat
Seated twist
Mid-Back
Extension
Ball squeezes

Day 23

Forward
punches
Aqua jogging
Arms curls
Standing water
push-ups

Day 24

The Basic Bridge
Side circles
Side-lying hip
bridges

Day 25

Wall Slides
Knee Curl
Quadriceps
stretch

Day 26

Step-Ups
Aqua jogging
Arms curls

Day 27

Reach back
Seated Marching
on the Spot
Mid-back
extension

Day 28

Single leg
deadlift
Quadriceps
stretch
Knee curls

Day 29

Lower Back
Stretch
Around the
Clock
Dumbbell Bench
Press

Day 30

Bird Dog
Leg Swings
Hamstring/Calf
Stretch

Day 31

Single-Leg
deadlifts
Rock the boat
Leg Swings

Day 32

Jog in place
Standing water
push-ups
Leg Lifts

Day 33

Reverse flyers
Seated mountain
pose
Single-Leg
Deadlifts

Day 34

Chest and Arm
Stretch
Back Leg Raise
Side Leg Raise

Day 35

Shoulder Rolls
Chair Dip
Sit to Stand

Day 36

Seated mountain
pose
Back Leg Raise
Reach back

Day 37

Forward
punches
Wrist radial
Lat Pull with
Band

Day 38

Thumb Flexion
Ball Squeezes
Forward
punches

Day 39

Qigong knee
rotation exercise
Hip extensions
Wall Angels

Day 40

Shoulder Stretch
Shoulder Shrug
Elbow flexion

Day 41

Overhead Reach
Lying hip
bridges
Foot slides

Day 42

Chest Squeeze
with Med Ball
Triceps stretch
Shoulder circles

Day 43

Step-Ups
Overhead stretch
Mermaid
Movement

Day 44

Lat Pull with
Band
Seated Twist
Shoulder and
Upper Back
Stretch

Day 45

Chest Stretch
Kneeling
Shoulder Tap
Push Up
Standing Side
Reach

Day 46	Day 47	Day 48	Day 49	Day 50
The Basic Bridge Leg Circles Lower Back Stretch	Tai Chi 24 Forms Movement Qigong Knee Rotation Exercise	Hip extension Knee Thrusters Ankle Circles	Hip Abductions Tai Chi 8 Forms Dumbbells Bench Press	Jog in a place Standing water push-ups Leg lifts
Day 51	**Day 52**	**Day 53**	**Day 54**	**Day 55**
Step-Ups Reverse Flyers Shoulder circles	Mermaid Movement Diagonal Shoulder Raise Pelvic tilt	Seated Mountain Pose Shoulder Press Lying Down Lying hip bridges	Hip extensions Chair Squat Rock the boat	Lat Pull with band Chest stretch Dumbbells Bench Press
Day 56	**Day 57**	**Day 58**	**Day 59**	**Day 60**
Chest and Arm Stretch Bicep curls Tai Chi 8 Forms Movement	Finger Marching Overhead Reach Elbow flexion	Mid-Back Extension Side circles Lying hip bridges	Forward punches Upright Rows Knee curls	Shoulder Shrug Neck Rotation Overhead stretch
Day 61	**Day 62**	**Day 63**	**Day 64**	**Day 65**
Quadriceps stretch Aqua jogging Water Arms curls	Step-Ups Diagonal Shoulder Raise Quadruped Opposite Arm and Leg Balance	Triceps extension Chest squeeze with Med Ball Standing Side Reach	Jog in a place Diagonal Shoulder Raise Pelvic tilt	Tai Chi 24 forms Elbows pronation Elbow Side Extensions
Day 66	**Day 67**	**Day 68**	**Day 69**	**Day 70**
Seated cow stretches Seated cat stretches Lower back stretch	Standing Side Reach Sit to stand Chair Squat	Mermaid Movement Shoulder rolls Shoulder stretch	Side Hip Raise Leg swings Wall Slides	Shoulder Press Lying Down Hip Abductions Basic bridge

Day 71	Day 72	Day 73	Day 74	Day 75
Tai Chi 8-Forms movement Seated Twist Seated Cow Stretch	Shoulder and Upper Back Stretch Standing Water Push-ups Leg Lifts	Step-Ups Back leg raise Bent knee raise	Triceps extension Assisted Finger Abductions Give the okay Make a "C"	Qigong knee rotation exercise Quadriceps stretch Knee curls

Day 76	Day 77	Day 78	Day 79	Day 80
Triceps extension Chair squat Seated chair twist	Mermaid Movement Tai Chi 8 forms	Quadruped Opposite Arm and Leg Balance Leg Swings Toe Raises	Finger Marching Triceps extension Overhead Reach	Lat Pull with Band Seated Twist

Day 81	Day 82	Day 83	Day 84	Day 85
Shoulder and Upper Back Stretch Quadruped Opposite Arm and Leg Balance	Ball Tap Side leg raise Around the clock	Kneeling Shoulder Tap Push Up The basic bridge Seated mountain pose	Finger Marching Give the okay Thumb flexion Wrist flexion	Step-Ups Wall push-ups Wrist stretches Chest squeeze with Med Ball

Day 86	Day 87	Day 88	Day 89	Day 90
Biceps curls Shoulder shrugs Forward punches	Leg swings One-legged Squat Ankle circles	Standing side reach Shoulder circles Upright rows	Forward punches Reach back Single-leg deadlift	Jog in a place Aqua jogging Standing water push-ups

Conclusion

Thank you for making it to the other end of this book. At this point, I'm sure that you have fully understood that as you grow older, an active life is more important than ever. Imagine how satisfying it would feel to move all your joints fluidly and without feeling any painful niggles that usually come with tight aging muscles and joints.

This book has equipped you with ALL the tools you need to not just regain your once-upon-a-time youthful strength but also to improve your flexibility, balance, and stability level in different parts of your upper and lower body. Kindly leave a review about what you think of this book.

Of course, there is a lot here to take in and do. But the primary key to your fitness growth and success is for you to keep it simple and stay consistent! Functional independence isn't regained in just a few days or weeks; you have to be resilient to get it! The best time to start was yesterday, but the second-best time is now!

I trust you will experience excellent health and well-being on the long road of life that lies before you and wish you my very best. Thank you for letting me share my knowledge with you.

Baz Thompson

References

Atkinson, D. (n.d.). Upper Arm Exercises You Can Do in the Pool. Retrieved from
https://primewomen.com/health/fitness/pool-arm-exercises/

Bowling, N. (2016). Wall Pushup Variations for A Strong Chest, Shoulders, and Back. Retrieved from
https://www.healthline.com/health/fitness-exercise/wall-pushups

Cordeau, B. (n.d.) How to Do: Lat Pulldown Loop Band. Retrieved from
https://www.skimble.com/exercises/41947-lat-pulldown-loop-band-how-to-do-exercise

East Wind Tai Chi Association. (n.d.). Tai Chi Forms. Retrieved from
http://www.itatkd.com/taichi-forms.html

Garofalo. M. P. (n.d.). Taijiquan 24 Form Yang Style. Retrieved from
https://www.egreenway.com/taichichuan/short.htm#Descriptions

Ghosh, A. (2017). Pilates for Seniors – The Complete Guide. Retrieved from
https://www.vivehealth.com/blogs/resources/pilates-for-seniors

Just Swim. (n.d.) Tone Your Body with Pool Edge Push-Ups. Retrieved from
https://www.swimming.org/justswim/pool-edge-push-ups/

Kenler, M. (2021) Banded Lat Pulldown: A Complete Guide | Form, Benefits & Alternatives. Retrieved from
https://www.anabolicaliens.com/blog/banded-lat-pulldown

Liang, H. (2015). Discover the Tai Chi 24 Forms. Retrieved from
https://ymaa.com/articles/2015/10/discover-the-tai-chi-24-form

Liang, H. (2016). Tai Chi 24-Form Movements. Retrieved from
https://ymaa.com/articles/2016/02/step-by-step-tai-chi-24-form

Lifeline. (n.d.). 14 Exercise for Seniors to Improve Strength and Balance. Retrieved from
https://www.lifeline.philips.com/resources/blog/2018/07/14-exercises-for-seniors-to-improve-strength-and-balance.html

Lindberg, S. (2020). Benefits of Jogging and Tips to Get Going. Retrieved from
https://www.healthline.com/health/aqua-jogging

Mansur, R. (2018). Do Bicep Curls for Seniors. Retrieved from
https://weight-training.wonderhowto.com/how-to/do-bicep-curls-for-seniors-254684/

More Life Health: Seniors. (n.d.) Bicep Curl Exercise. Retrieved from
https://morelifehealth.com/bicep-curls

Nurse Next Door. (2020). 6 Easy and Safe Exercises for Seniors. Retrieved from
https://www.nursenextdoor.com/blog/6-easy-and-safe-exercises-for-seniors/

Occhipinti, A. (2018). 3 Pilates Exercises to Help Seniors Improve Balance & Mobility. Retrieved from
https://www.afpafitness.com/blog/pilates-exercises-help-seniors-improve-balance-mobility

Ogle, M. (2020). How to Do Mermaid Sides Stretch in Pilates: Proper Form, Variations, and Common Mistakes.
Retrieved from
https://www.verywellfit.com/learn-mermaid-side-stretch-2704698

Ogle, M. (2020). How to Do Single Leg Circle in Pilates: Proper Form, Variations, and Common Mistakes. Retrieved
from
https://www.verywellfit.com/how-to-do-one-leg-circle-2704673

Pizer, A. (2020) How to Do Cat-Cow Stretch (Chakravakasana) in Yoga. Retrieved from
https://www.verywellfit.com/cat-cow-stretch-chakravakasana-3567178

Qiyas. (n.d.). Best Pool Exercises for Seniors: Legs, Knee, Arms, Core. Retrieved from
https://hydroactive.ca/pool-exercises-for-seniors/

Ratini, M. (2020). 10 Ways to Exercise Hands and Fingers. Retrieved from
https://www.webmd.com/osteoarthritis/ss/slideshow-hand-finger-exercises

Schrift, D. (n.d.) Upper Arm Exercise for Seniors and The Elderly. Retrieved from
https://eldergym.com/upper-arm-exercises/

Senior Lifestyles. (n.d.) Infographic: Top 10 Chair Yoga Position for Seniors. Retrieved from
https://www.seniorlifestyle.com/resources/blog/infographic-top-10-chair-yoga-positions-for-seniors/

Shillington, P. (2017). Never Too Late: Building Muscles and Strength After 60. Retrieved from
https://baptisthealth.net/baptist-health-news/never-late-building-muscle-strength-60/

Shou-Yu, L. (2012). Learning Tai Chi – The 24 and 48 Forms. Retrieved from
https://ymaa.com/articles/learning-tai-chi-the-24-and-48-forms

Talk Early, Talk Often. (n.d.). Exercise for Senior Citizens: Try Triceps Extensions for Aging Fitness. Retrieved from
http://www.talk-early-talk-often.com/exercise-for-senior-citizens.html

The Middletown Home. (n.d.). The Benefits of Tai Chi for Seniors. Retrieved from
https://middletownhome.org/tai-chi-benefits-seniors/

Tummee. (n.d.). Chair Seated Twists. Retrieved from
https://www.tummee.com/yoga-poses/chair-seated-twists

Waehner, P. (2019). Total Body Strength Workout for Seniors. Retrieved from
https://www.verywellfit.com/total-body-strength-workout-for-seniors-1230958

Williams, L. (2020). How to Do a Side Lateral Raise: Proper Form, Variations, and Common Mistakes. Retrieved from
https://www.verywellfit.com/side-lateral-raise-4588211

Willhoite, J. (2020). Punching Bag Workout Tips for Seniors Stress Relief. Retrieved from
https://seniorslifestylemag.com/health-well-being/punching-bag-workout-tips-for-senior-stress-relief/